Rosemary Conley's
New Inch Loss Plan

ARROW

First published in 1998

1 3 5 7 9 10 8 6 4 2

Copyright © Rosemary Conley Enterprises, 1998

The right of Rosemary Conley to be identified as the author of this
work has been asserted by her in accordance with the Copyright,
Designs and Patents Act, 1988

First published in the United Kingdom in 1998
by Arrow Books Limited
Random House UK Ltd
20 Vauxhall Bridge Road, London SW1V 2SA

Random House Australia (Pty) Limited
20 Alfred Street, Milsons Point, Sydney,
New South Wales 2061, Australia

Random House New Zealand Limited
18 Poland Road, Glenfield,
Auckland 10, New Zealand

Random House South Africa (Pty) Limited
Endulini, 5a Jubilee Road, Parktown 2193, South Africa

Random House UK Limited Reg. No. 954009

ISBN 0 09 927102 8

Designed by Roger Walker

Typeset in Giovanni and Frutiger

Printed and bound in Great Britain by
Butler & Tanner Ltd, Frome and London

IMPORTANT

If you have a medical condition or are pregnant, the diet and exercises described in this book should not be followed without first
consulting your doctor. All guidelines and warnings should be
read carefully, and the author and publisher cannot accept respon-
sibility for injuries or damage arising out of a failure to comply
with the same.

Contents

Acknowledgements

As my professional life gets busier and busier I rely more and more on my wonderful team who endlessly endeavour to ease my workload. This book would not have been possible without the help of my PA, Louise Cowell, and my assistant, Melody Patterson, who coped with my scribblings and directions and put them into a legible format before the book was sent to my editor.

The creation of 28 workouts was a major task and very time-consuming. Mary Morris is Training and Development Manager for Rosemary Conley Diet & Fitness Clubs and so willingly works right alongside me, making sure that all my exercises are technically correct at the same time as being as supremely effective as possible. Thank you Mary for your skill, patience and dedication to ensuring this exercise plan will really work for everyone who does it.

Thanks must also go to Alan Olley for taking the photographs with his usual expertise; to Dennis Barker, Art Director, for his input; and to designer Roger Walker for designing the book so that the contents appear in an easy-to-follow way.

None of my books would ever reach the bookstands without the help of all these people, but particular thanks must go to Jan Bowmer. Jan has edited my work for the last ten years and her enthusiasm, encouragement and attention to detail has helped me to create books that, hopefully, change people's eating and exercise habits for the better – and for life.

A note from the author

My original Inch Loss Plan was published in 1990 and it became a firm favourite with hundreds of thousands of people. Even now, people turn up at roadshows or book-signing opportunities and bring along their rather old and dog-eared copy for me to sign. Today, so much more is known about how the body works and how to exercise it to maximum effect. My knowledge has increased enormously, and I am now delighted to bring you a revised and updated version of that original huge bestseller. The diet is as effective as ever, with some more recent additions incorporating foods that are currently available in supermarkets and food stores to offer greater variety. The exercises have been updated to incorporate the very latest advice and techniques to enable you to enjoy maximum benefits to your body.

The positive thoughts of the day that are included in this new book have not changed from my earlier book, because the philosophy they contain is, I believe, ageless. Many people have told me how they have taken on board the ideas and suggestions from the Inch Loss Plan and have changed their lives for the better as a result. I am so grateful to the many thousands of people who have written to tell me how my diet and exercises have not only helped them to transform their shape but also brought huge benefits to their health. It is very exciting.

Introduction

In just 28 days from now would you like to be the proud owner of a new body? Would you also like to be in control of your emotions and on the path to a highly successful future? In other words, become a new you. If it sounds too good to be true, I assure you it's not. In just one month you can dramatically improve the shape of your body by losing weight, burning fat and toning up your muscles. The bonus of all of this is that your confidence will also improve. With increased confidence, you will find all kinds of opportunities that previously you wouldn't have had the self-esteem to even consider. So how is all this going to happen? Simply by following the day-by-day eating, exercise and positive thinking programme that is detailed in this book. You will never again be labelled or label yourself a failure.

It is so much more fun being a winner than a loser, and if you think of yourself as a born loser, you are wrong! In fact the only things you are going to lose from now on are weight and inches!

Conquering your weight problem is probably the most important thing in your life right now. No doubt you are among the many who seem to have tried every diet around only to find that they just don't work. Actually, most diets do work, it's only our willpower that fails! So how can we get more willpower? Since we can't just purchase it from the chemist's, we have to manufacture our own incentive. Encouragement and real results are the essential ingredients required to nurture adequate supplies of willpower and to keep it growing. If we have no reason to slim, if no one cares whether we slim or not, or if we feel we are trying hard on a diet but nothing seems to be happening, no wonder we get fed up. All these negative influences convince us we are diet failures. Have you ever said, 'I think I was meant to be big' or 'I only have to look at a cream cake and I gain 2lb' or even 'I can't diet'? These are all negative statements that you have imprinted on to your brain. As long as you still think these thoughts you will believe them and you won't succeed. So how do you turn these 'I can't' messages around to positive 'I can and I will' statements? You need a time limit which is short enough to be attractive but long enough to effect a result. Twenty-eight days is perfect. If you are going to make this real effort for 28 days, not only do you want to quantify the difference on the bathroom scales, you also want to actually see the difference in the mirror and on the tape measure. You probably want to reduce by at least one dress size, if not two! You want to wear some of those clothes in the wardrobe that you haven't been able to wear for ages. You want to really look a lot slimmer, and this will happen. You definitely don't want to go hungry or eat 'rabbit food' all the time, and you don't want to mess around counting calories. You would like some freedom in what you eat and drink. Yes, and you probably would like an alcoholic drink, too. I know this sounds too good to be true but it can be done.

The diet in this New Inch Loss Plan is based on low-fat eating of around 1,400 calories a day for women (men can increase the quantities by 25 per cent). Each day you are allowed 450ml ($\frac{3}{4}$ pint) of milk to add to your breakfast cereal, tea or coffee or to use to make sauces such as parsley sauce or desserts such as rice pudding or custard. In addition, women are allowed 1 unit of alcohol per day, while men can enjoy 2 units. There is great freedom of choice in the menus listed so that you can design the diet to suit you. You don't have to eat the recommended menu for any specific day. You can substitute any breakfast, lunch and dinner menu included in this book. I know only too well that for a diet to work it has to fit in with an individual's taste and daily routine.

Now what about exercise? Few people enjoy jogging or pumping iron in the local gym three evenings a week, so I've got over that problem too. Just 15 minutes a day is all that is required initially, and in the comfort and convenience of your own home. The exercises are easy to do and combine fat-burning aerobic activity with muscle-toning strength exercises to improve your shape. You will enjoy your workout more if you do the exercises to music, so select your favourite tracks and make your workout a truly enjoyable experience.

Each week you will have 2 rest days. This is to allow your energy stores to stock up and to give you a greater level of fitness as you progress. On your rest days you can stay active, but you certainly shouldn't work to the point of exhaustion. If you do, your energy levels will drop rather than increase.

This exercise programme is progressive and by Week 4 you will be working your body quite hard, with enormous effect. This effect will be enhanced by the fact that you will have worked towards it gradually. The benefits to your muscles will have been achieved without discomfort or pain, and certainly without injury. This will then set you up for a fit and healthy body that you can maintain for the rest of your life.

If you have a lot of weight to lose, then at the end of the 28 days you can continue with the diet and exercises. The diet is perfectly safe and effective for you to follow until you reach your goal weight. Many people will also gain enormous benefits from attending a Rosemary Conley Diet & Fitness Club class. At that class you will be shown exercises similar to those in this book and will be given diet and fitness advice by qualified instructors. For more details see the back of the book.

Use this book as your friend. Read it daily and if you follow the advice that it gives you, I promise you that it will change your life.

How it all began

If this is the first of my books that you have read, you may be interested to hear how I discovered the benefits of low-fat eating. (If you already know the story, you can skip this section and turn to page 12 to continue.)

In 1986, I was forced on to a very-low-fat diet for health reasons, because I had a gall bladder that grumbled very painfully when I ate fatty food. As I didn't want to undergo the inconvenience of surgery to remove the offending gall bladder, I opted for very-low-fat eating, with the miraculous side effect of acquiring slim hips and thighs for the first time in my adult life. Some years earlier, I had lost almost 2st (12.7kg) from my heaviest weight of 10st 3lb (65kg), but I still had ugly hips and thighs. All other efforts to lose fat from the offending areas proved a disaster, because if I lost weight below 8st 7lb (54kg), my bust disappeared, yet nothing went from my legs or posterior! That was unshiftable, or so I thought! My exercise class students witnessed the low fat diet's remarkable effect on my body – I had lost only 6lb (2.7kg) but all from my problem areas – and then they tried the diet and reaped similar benefits.

Further extensive trials were carried out before my first Hip and Thigh Diet was published in 1988. Such was the response from readers who wrote to me with their amazing success stories, that it was decided I should write an extended version of the book, and the Complete Hip and Thigh Diet was published in 1989. Total sales to date exceed two million. Why? Simply because it works! Low-fat eating

leads to a leaner body, and that's all we really ask of a diet, isn't it?

Years ago, I used to be obsessed about my weight problem. I didn't know where to turn and I felt really desperate. I have struggled with my weight ever since, because I adore food and have a large appetite. But I am not a 'diet prisoner' any more. Now I am free to eat lovely food – lots of lovely food! I never go hungry. In fact, at every mealtime, I eat until I feel full. I do not have to count calories all the time and I eat three meals a day. But I eat only food that is low in fat, I don't eat between meals and I've stopped bingeing. I don't need to binge any more – I can have plenty to eat at mealtimes. Now this hasn't happened just to me. My low-fat eating programme, detailed in my Hip and Thigh Diet books and other books I have written, has helped hundreds of thousands of overweight men and women to lose weight and inches from their problem areas for the first time in their lives! I have received literally thousands of letters from readers telling me of their successes. It has been so rewarding for me to read about the happiness and freedom from the prison of obesity that is now enjoyed by so many. This is a typical letter:

Dear Rosemary,
I know you must receive hundreds of letters like mine, but I have been meaning to write to you now for ages. I am a trained nurse and I've always had a weight problem. My hips and thighs have always been bulky, making me feel uncomfortable in trousers or tight jeans. I am 23 and for the past three years I have been piling on the pounds without realising it, until I finally took a good look at myself weighing in at 12st 3lb (77.5kg) at 5ft 4in (1.6m).

As a nurse I knew it was unhealthy to be so over-weight and I felt extremely unhappy with what I had become. I knew I had bad eating habits when I started secretly to buy sweets from several different shops and ensure the wrappers were well hidden from my boyfriend. Then I started to make myself vomit and knew I had a problem. I had always been an erratic binge eater and was forever on a diet without losing weight, due to bingeing/starving/vomiting. I would always be 'starting the diet tomorrow' and I would eat everything in sight until I could hardly move. My boyfriend knew nothing of these habits, and the first move was to tell him. It gave me incredible relief actually to admit to someone how unhappy I was with these eating habits.

Just after Christmas, we decided to get married, so I had until June to slim down. I was already feeling depressed about having to diet and I hadn't heard of yours. First, I tried the Cambridge Diet, which just did not work for me. I had tried it before and put on more weight because I didn't re-educate my eating habits, but I needed to see immediate results to get the enthusiasm to continue dieting. Next, I tried the 3-day diet which was so depriving during the diet days (3 days on, 2 days off) that I still binged every week, felt terrible mentally and my weight fluctuated! Then I bought your book. I was most sceptical when reading all the letters, thinking it must be 'fixed'. My boyfriend commented that surely I couldn't lose weight eating so much food! I started the diet on April 16th and by June 30th (my wedding day) I had lost 21lb (9.5 kg) – all from areas previously unshiftable! I couldn't believe how healthy I felt. I no longer craved sweet things, no longer felt the need to binge and have only cheated twice (and I mean one chocolate – not the whole box as before).

As a nurse, I cannot think of a healthier diet to follow and can see no disadvantages in it. I feel fully satisfied appetite-wise and have lost weight easily, despite having bread or rice every day. I looked my slimmest ever on my wedding day and thoroughly enjoyed my holiday. I have never in my life looked forward to starting a diet, but by the end of my holiday I couldn't wait to get back on it to maintain my slimmer figure (with every other diet, I have put weight back on and more!). I have a new wardrobe full of clothes I couldn't wear before, and now fit comfortably into a size 10/12 instead of struggling into a size 14. I've lost 4in (10cm) all over, and my friends cannot believe it – they have all been buying your book! I feel so glad that I've finally found something that works and am not confined to a life of bingeing/vomiting, etc. I can go out for the odd meal without suffering from the binge factor because we had a dessert. I've recommended your diet to various patients, as I don't see how anyone can fail to benefit from a low-fat diet. I feel I owe you so much because this diet has changed my life.

Yours sincerely,
Belinda Robinson

Almost a thousand readers completed a questionnaire after following my Hip and Thigh Diet. This gave me a vast amount of information about their needs and desires. Their comments were so interesting and helpful in enabling me to arrive at a diet plan perfected for absolute maximum effect. Men have trimmed their tums without losing their physiques. Women have whittled away their waistlines, flattened their tummies and shed their child-bearing hips and jodhpur thighs but have held on to their bustlines.

I've tried to learn from readers' comments and, hopefully, have arrived at the ideal blend of appetite satisfaction combined with gastro-nomic appeal. In other words, if you look for-ward to your next meal and feel happy and full after the last one, you're unlikely to cheat and have a binge. Furthermore, if you can become satisfied with your regular daily bread, you will get into a new routine which will take you on a continuing journey of successful weight maintenance.

After appearing on a television programme in Scotland, I was asked by an eminent professor of physiology to try to establish the long-term success of my Hip and Thigh Diet slimmers. As I was sending a copy of the new book to all those slimmers who were mentioned in my Complete Hip and Thigh Diet, I decided to include with it a second questionnaire. I asked for details of how well they had maintained their new figures or if, in fact, they hadn't. I issued 83 Maintenance Questionnaires, and 59 were returned. Of those, only 2 people had regained a significant amount of their lost weight. If we look on the black side and assume that the remaining 24 readers who did not reply had regained their weight, it still left over two-thirds who had maintained their lost weight. This meant that almost 70 per cent had actually maintained their new figures. This was an incredible result, bearing in mind the general statistics of 98 per cent failure rates reported for most dieting attempts. The professor was impressed.

So why did the Hip and Thigh Diet work when previous diets didn't? Why did it sell so many copies by word of mouth? Why did fol-lowers of the diet maintain their new figures instead of regaining their old ones? The answer is simply that they enjoyed it. It didn't seem like a diet – in fact, if there was one sentence that kept reappearing in most of the letters I received, it was: 'You can't call this a diet, it's more a way of eating.' And if we can enjoy a reducing diet, it follows that we won't mind following the basic principles in the long term. But in reality, it is even easier than that because we do actually, amazingly, lose the taste for very fatty foods. Bread tastes wonderful without butter, potatoes are delicious without fat, we can eat spaghetti, rice and porridge – all with a clear conscience. That's the secret – freedom.

Now this freedom in our eating habits has been complemented with a programme of exercises that actually does something beneficial for both your health and your figure. Additionally, there are a few lessons in positive thinking that will effectively change the way you look at yourself, as well as those around you. In fact, your whole life is going to change so much for the better, you will be amazed! From now on, if you follow this 28-day New Inch Loss Plan, you should achieve heights you didn't even know existed for you. I promise you've got absolutely nothing to lose but your inches. Have fun and enjoy the results!

Diet and Exercise Instructions

THE DIET

It is very important that you weigh and measure yourself at the beginning of the day on which you commence the New Inch Loss Plan. Enter the details on the Weight and Inch Loss Record Chart at the back of this book.

Select one breakfast, lunch and dinner menu each day, except on the 7th, 14th, 21st and 28th days (designed to be Sundays) when you should choose a breakfast, lunch and supper menu. However, you are welcome to change the timing of the menus to suit your individual routine. For instance, you could have your main meal at lunchtime and your snack meal in the evening.

It is important for you to enjoy your menus and feel satisfied. If you find a favourite menu one day, select it again if you wish. Menus may be interchanged to suit your individual taste.

Each day offers two choices at each mealtime, including a vegetarian option. Because there is usually less protein in vegetarian dishes, more yogurt has been included in these menus to compensate for this. If for any reason you are unable to eat milk, yogurt or cottage cheese, it is essential that you take a calcium supplement. As egg yolks are high in fat, limit your consumption to 2 per week (vegetarians can eat 3).

The menus listed should satisfy your appetite. Ideally, you should eat all that has been suggested at each mealtime. But don't force the food down if you are adequately satisfied with less. However, if you still feel you need to eat more, fill up with extra vegetables to satisfy your natural appetite. It is important to eat enough to prevent you from feeling hungry between meals. If you do feel hunger pangs, nibble on carrot, celery or cucumber sticks or sliced green peppers. Do not eat anything else between meals.

Use this diet to re-educate your eating pattern, and your appetite, towards three meals a day. It is a really good habit to learn. If you eat sufficient at each mealtime, you shouldn't need anything for later on!

There is no restriction on the amount of non-alcoholic drinks you consume, but all cold drinks should be low-calorie brands, and tea and coffee should be drunk black or with milk from your allowance. Use an artificial sweetener in place of sugar whenever possible. Alcoholic drinks should be restricted to 1 per day for women and 2 for men unless otherwise stated.

Observe and learn the list of foods to avoid listed on page 13. These are high in fat and should be eliminated during the course of the New Inch Loss Plan. During the 28-day Programme try to stick strictly to the menus listed within the diet.

Diet Notes

- Bread should be wholemeal whenever possible. For guidance, 1 slice of regular bread from a large thin-sliced loaf weighs 25g (1oz). A slice from a large medium-sliced loaf weighs 40g (1½oz). Unless otherwise specified in the menus, 1 slice equals 25g (1oz). 'Light bread' means low-calorie brands such as Nimble or St Michael Lite Bread.
- 'Diet yogurt' means any low-fat or fat-free brand (1 × 150g/5oz pot should contain no more than 70 kcals). All fromage frais and cottage cheese should also be low-fat brands.
- Gravy may be taken with the dinner menus, provided it is made with gravy powder or low-fat granules. Do not add meat juices from the roasting tin unless you first discard the fat.
- 'One piece of fresh fruit' means 1 average apple, orange etc., or 115g (4oz) any fresh fruit.
- Pasta and rice are restricted to 50g (2oz) dry weight per portion unless otherwise specified. 50g (2oz) dry weight rice weighs 150g (5oz)

when cooked, and 50g (2oz) dry weight pasta weighs 175g (6oz). Choose wholemeal varieties where possible. Always boil without adding oil or fat. Unlimited quantities of tinned or fresh beansprouts may be added to bulk up small quantities of rice.

- 'Unlimited vegetables' includes all vegetables, except potatoes, providing they are cooked and served without fat.

Sauces and Dressings

The following may be consumed freely:

Brown sauce
Chilli sauce
Fat-free salad dressings
Horseradish sauce
Lemon juice
Marmite
Mint sauce
Mustard
Oil-free vinaigrette
Soy sauce
Tomato ketchup
Vinegar (any type)
Worcester sauce

For other sauces and dressings check the nutrition panel on the label before you buy and only select those with 4 per cent or less fat, except for items of which you will consume only minimal amounts.

Foods to avoid

The following foods are strictly forbidden while you are following the diet, unless they are specifically included in the diet menus or recipes or contain 4 per cent or less fat. Exceptions are made only for vegetarians who may include a little low-fat cheese and a few drops of oil in their cooking.

Avocado pears and olives
Butter, margarine, low-fat spreads, mayonnaise
Cakes, biscuits, pastries, quiches, egg custard, crackers, marzipan, sponge puddings etc.
Cheese: all varieties including low-fat brands, except cottage cheese
Chocolate, toffees, fudge, caramel, butterscotch
Cream, cream cheese, soured cream
Crisps and snacks
Desserts made from cream, such as crème brûlée, crème caramel, home-made ice-cream
Dressings and sauces containing more than 4 per cent fat
Fats and oils, e.g. cooking oil, olive oil, lard, dripping, suet, fat from meat
Fatty meats, e.g. goose
Fried foods of any kind (except dry-fried)
Full-fat yogurts, Greek yogurt (check the label for fat content)
Horlicks, drinking chocolate, cocoa and cocoa products
Lemon curd, peanut butter, chocolate spread
Meat products such as Scotch eggs, pork pies, faggots, black pudding, haggis, pâté, salami, sausages, skin from all meats and poultry

Daily Allowance

In addition to the menus listed you may consume each day:

150ml (1/4 pint) unsweetened fruit juice, any flavour
450ml (3/4 pint) skimmed or semi-skimmed milk
1 measure of alcoholic drink (2 for men). 1 measure = 1 single gin or 300ml (1/2 pint) beer or lager or 1 glass of wine or sherry.

Note
All branded products included in this book were available at the time of going to press, but manufacturers' ranges are subject to change. Vegetarians should also check the list of ingredients, as manufacturers' recipes may change.

The Exercises

This exercise programme is specifically designed to help you lose inches and tone and tighten all those areas that concern you so that you can achieve the shape you want. It is now known that regular exercise is the best way to lose inches and at the same time achieve optimum health. Any exercise that gets you out of breath draws upon the excess fat stored on your body, and if you follow a programme of regular exercise – and keep it up – you will see a significant inch loss. Add in some vital muscle-toning exercises which make each individual muscle work hard, and the result will be a body finely tuned to cope with the demands of daily life. It will also enable you to acquire a better shape than you ever thought possible. This programme offers all the tools you need to achieve this, and in just 4 weeks!

HOW THE EXERCISE PROGRAMME WORKS

This programme becomes progressively more challenging by gradually increasing the amount of time that you exercise for and making each exercise you perform more intense. For example, in Week 1 you will do your toning exercises for about only 3 minutes and perform just a few repetitions of each one, but by Week 4 you'll be spending 7 minutes on the toning exercises, with more exercises and each one becoming significantly harder to perform. The same happens for each part of the workout so that the overall session time of 15 minutes in Week 1 doubles to 30 minutes by Week 4.

Over a period of 7 days you will actually only exercise on 5 of them. This complies with the current guidelines laid down by the Health Education Authority, which recommends exercising for 30 minutes, 5 times a week. It is important to have 2 days free from exercise each week in order to re-fuel the body properly. Since the diet is high in carbohydrates, you will be taking in sufficient fuel to prepare you for each day, but if you were to continue to exercise without taking any rest days you would feel progressively more tired.

GOLDEN RULES FOR EXERCISING

- It is important that you listen to your body and only do as much as is comfortable. If the progression of intensity is too much for you, then simply stay on the same level as the previous day, or even the previous week, until you feel able to do more.
- Always wear layers of loose and comfortable clothing so that you can remove items as you

become warmer. A T-shirt and leggings are ideal, and it is important to wear supportive and cushioned exercise shoes to prevent undue stress on your joints.

- Have a glass of water close by so that you can stay well-hydrated as you exercise. The body is more efficient at burning fat if you keep taking in plenty of fluid, particularly during hot weather. Also try not to work out in a very warm room, as this will cause you to dehydrate more quickly. In the colder months, it's a good idea to turn down your central heating while you exercise.
- If possible, exercise to your favourite music. The best pace is one you can comfortably march to and then you know it will fit most of the programme. At the end of each workout, put on some slow, relaxing music to help you wind down as you perform the cool-down stretches.

WHERE WILL YOU LOSE THOSE INCHES ?

As long as you combine this exercise programme with low-fat eating you will lose inches from those areas that concern you the most. For example, if you are a pear shape and carry most of your fat around your hips and thighs, then you will see a real improvement in that area very quickly, since this is where you have large fat deposits. And performing the aerobic section on

each day that you exercise will ensure you are doing the best type of activity to burn off excess fat from those areas. Be aware, though, that you will lose fat and inches from around your whole body. This is when those toning exercises become so important, because if you have an area of the body that does not carry much excess fat, it is vital that you work on the muscle there to give tone and shape to that area. By repeatedly making an individual muscle work hard, you increase the amount of muscle in that area, and this helps to provide a balanced shape to your body. For example, if you carry fat mostly on the hips and thighs, then performing plenty of upper body toning exercises will give you this balanced result.

SEEING RESULTS

The more inches you have to lose, the quicker you will see results. Combining the exercise programme with the low-fat eating plan will enable you to see encouraging results almost immediately, and by the end of the Week 4 you will be amazed at what you have achieved in such a short time. You will have more energy and be slimmer and fitter too. Take 3 photographs of yourself at the beginning of this programme – a front view, a side view and a back view. Then take them again after 28 days – and see the difference!

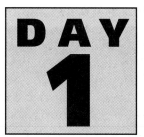

DAY 1

Today is going to have a greater significance on your life than you could ever imagine. You are about to begin an eating plan that will both satisfy your appetite and reduce the amount of fat on your body. You are also about to embark on a series of exercises that will start you on the road to a more beautiful body – a body of which you will be proud. Your body may have become out of shape through general neglect over a period of years, yet you can transform it incredibly in a matter of weeks with this healthy diet and safe and effective exercise plan. You don't have to starve or wear yourself out jogging for miles. You'll achieve much more by using this effective eating plan and fat-burning aerobic workout and toning exercises, and the programme will soon become a way of life.

The warm-up exercises wake up your body, mobilise your joints and prepare your muscles for action. They encourage better posture and promote a sense of wellbeing.

Posture is particularly important to the way we look. If the body is in correct alignment, it works efficiently. Poor posture, on the other hand, results in unnecessary stresses and strains which can have serious effects on our health. So, today, please make a special effort to concentrate on your posture all day! Pull that tummy right in and stand tall with shoulders back and down. Get into the habit of having a good posture.

Find yourself a tight skirt or pair of trousers or jeans that you can hardly do up! Use this as your measuring garment and try it on at 3-day intervals to see the improvement.

—Menu—

BREAKFAST

25g (1oz) bran flakes plus a medium-sized banana, sliced, served with milk from allowance and 1 teaspoon brown sugar

OR

40g (1½oz) wholemeal toast spread with 2 teaspoons marmalade, plus 150g (5oz) diet yogurt, any flavour

LUNCH

2 slices of wholemeal bread spread with mustard, pickle or reduced-oil salad dressing, and filled with 50g (2oz) wafer thin chicken, and unlimited lettuce, tomatoes and cucumber

OR

Jacket potato (any size) topped with 115g (4oz) baked beans, plus 1 × 150g (5oz) diet yogurt, any flavour

DINNER

175g (6oz) chicken joint (weighed with bone) with all skin removed or 75g (3oz) red meat (no fat), served with unlimited vegetables, including potatoes
PLUS
MELON SURPRISE (see recipe, page 179)
OR
VEGETABLE KEBABS (see recipe, page 184)
PLUS
CHEESE PEARS (see recipe, page 175)

WEEK 1: TIME: 15 MINUTES

5	5	3	2
WARM UP	AEROBIC	TONE	STRETCH

WARM UP – MOBILITY

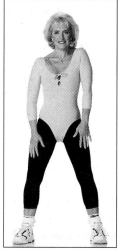

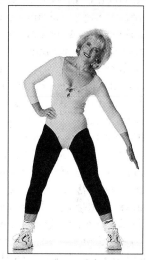

1 Alternate Shoulder Lifts Stand tall with feet apart, head up and shoulders back. Now lift alternate shoulders up and down. Do 12, changing sides each time.

2 Side Bends With feet apart and knees slightly bent, gently lean to one side, keeping the hips still and reaching out with one arm. Lift up and do the same to the other side. Repeat 6 times to each side.

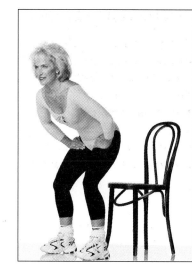

3 Knee Bends With legs wider than shoulder-width apart and feet turned out slightly, bend your knees in line with the toes, taking your hips back as if you were trying to sit in a chair. Come up without locking the knees fully. Repeat 6 times slowly.

4 March on the Spot
Standing tall, with head up and shoulders back, march on the spot, allowing your arms to swing naturally. Make sure the heels land on the floor each time. March for 2 minutes.

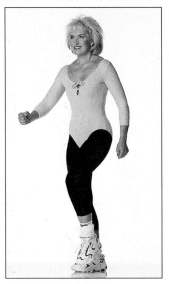

6 Calf Stretch
Hold on to the back of a chair and place one foot in front of the other, with the front leg bent and the back leg straight. Lean towards the front leg slightly and check that both feet point forward. Hold for 6 seconds, then change legs and repeat.

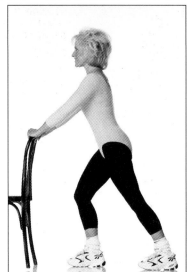

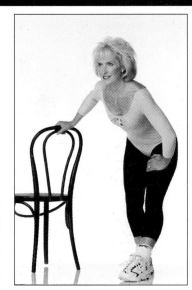

7 Back of Thigh Stretch Stand side-on to a chair and hold on to it for support. Bend the leg nearest to the chair and keep the other leg straight, with your hand on the thigh. Now lean forward, keeping your head in line and your back straight, until you feel a stretch in the back of the thigh. Hold for 6 seconds, then turn around to change legs and repeat.

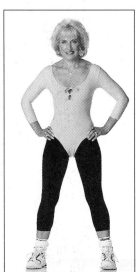

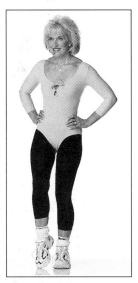

8 Front of Thigh Stretch Still standing side-on to the chair, take hold of the outside leg around the ankle and bend the supporting knee slightly. Keep the knees together and push the outside hip forward to feel a stretch down the front of the thigh. Hold for 6 seconds, then turn around to change legs, and repeat.

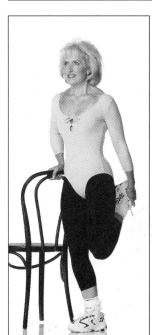

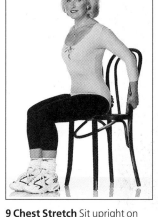

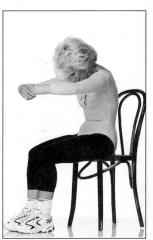

9 Chest Stretch Sit upright on the edge of the chair, with feet flat on the floor. Take your hands behind you to hold the back of the chair, and feel a stretch across the chest. Hold for 6 seconds.

10 Upper Back Stretch Still sitting on the chair, bring your arms in front at chest height and drop your head forward. Now push your hands away from the upper back and hold for 6 seconds.

5 Step Touch Take a step out to the right and bring the left toe to the right foot, then immediately step back to the left. Keep stepping from side to side rhythmically, bending your knees as the feet come together. Take 32 steps.

SEQUENCE 1

11a Step Touch Stand tall, with your hands on your hips, and take a step out to the side with the right foot. Now tap the left foot close to the right foot and immediately step to the left, tapping the right foot to the left. Keep changing sides, bending your knees as the feet come together. Perform 8 times, then change to 11b.

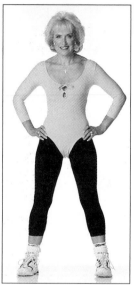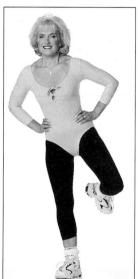

11b Hopscotch Take a step out to the right and bend your left heel up behind you, then step out to the left, bringing the right heel up. Repeat 8 times, then go back to 11a.

Repeat this sequence 4 times.

SEQUENCE 2

12a Double Side Steps Now take 2 steps out to the right and then back to the left. Make sure the whole foot makes contact with the floor and keep your tummy in and your back straight. Perform twice through, then change to 12b.

12b Walk Forward and Back Step forward on the right leg and continue moving forward for 3 steps, and on the 4th count bring the left foot to tap to the right foot and clap your hands. Now step back with the left foot for 3 steps and on the 4th count bring the right foot to tap to the left foot and clap your hands. Repeat twice through before going back to 12a.

Repeat this sequence 4 times.

SEQUENCE 3

13a Box Step This exercise has 4 counts. Take a step forward on the right foot, as if to the top right corner of a box (count 1). Now bring the left foot out to the top left corner (count 2). Step back again with the right (count 3) and follow with the left (count 4).

Complete 4 full box steps before changing to 13b.

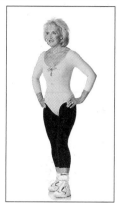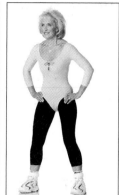
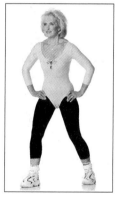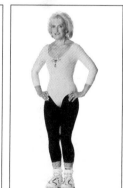

13b Half Jacks Now tap the ball of the right foot out to the side. Bring the feet together and tap the left foot out. Keep changing sides, making sure you keep the knee of the supporting leg slightly bent and stand tall throughout. Repeat 8 times before going back to 13a.

Repeat this sequence 4 times.

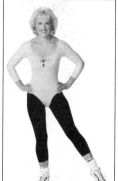

This whole aerobics session should last for around 5 minutes.

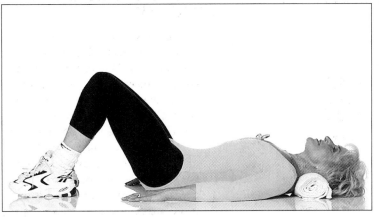

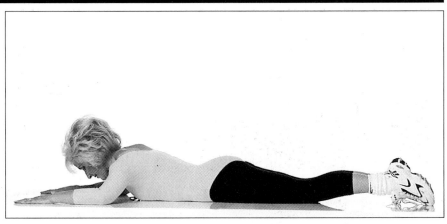

14 Pelvic Tilt Lie on your back, with knees bent and feet flat on the floor. Place a rolled-up towel under your head to reduce tension on the neck. Now pull your tummy in tight so that the whole of the spine touches the floor (you will feel the pelvis tilt naturally), then release. Perform 4 times slowly and under control, breathing out as you pull in and breathing in as you release. Rest and repeat.

15 Back Raises Lie on your tummy, with your arms out in front and the elbows bent. Now gently raise your upper body from the floor, keeping the whole of the forearms on the floor. Look down at the floor all the time so that the neck stays long. Repeat 4 times, then rest and repeat.

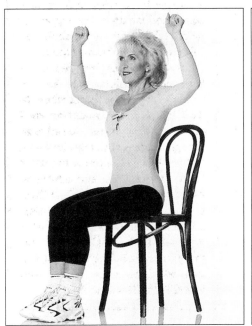

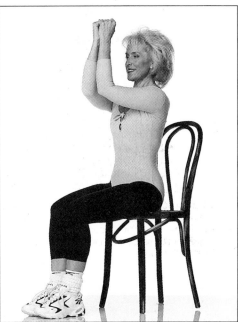

16 Chest Toner Sitting towards the edge of a chair, with your feet flat on the floor, bring your arms out to the sides so that each arm forms a 90-degree angle at chest height. Now squeeze the elbows towards each other, keeping them in line with the chest. Breathe out as you bring them in, and breathe in as you open them again. Perform slowly and smoothly 6 times, then rest and repeat.

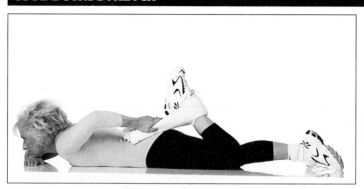

17 Front of Thigh Stretch Lie on your front, with your hands resting under your chin. Now, using your right hand, take hold of the right ankle (you can use a towel to assist if you find this difficult). Bring the heel close to the hip and push the hip down gently into the floor. Hold for 10 seconds, then change legs and repeat.

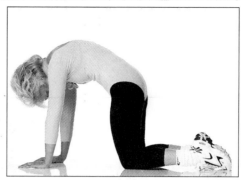

18 Spine Stretch Come up into a box shape on hands and knees. Now pull your tummy in tightly, arching your back and tucking your hips under. Breathe normally. Hold for 8 seconds, then release.

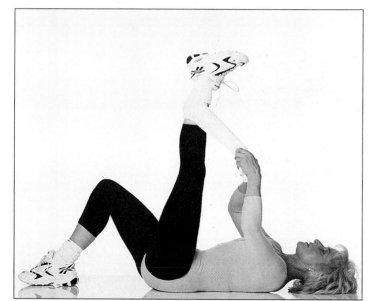

19 Back of Thigh Stretch Lie on your back, with knees bent and feet flat on the floor. Now take hold behind one leg, using a towel to assist, and ease the leg towards the chest. Try to keep the leg as straight as possible, with both hips remaining on the floor, to feel a stretch at the back of the thigh. Hold for 10 seconds, then change legs and repeat.

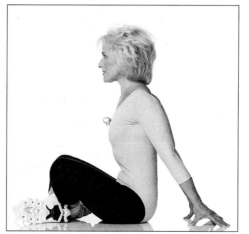

20 Chest Stretch Sitting cross-legged, with your back straight and your head up, take both hands behind you on the floor and pull your shoulder blades together at the back to feel a stretch across the chest. Hold for 8 seconds.

POSITIVE THOUGHT FOR THE DAY

This diet will work if you follow it. These exercises will reshape your body if you do them. The proportion of fat deposited on your body will reduce in a most dramatic way in the next 4 weeks. The fat we eat becomes fat on our bodies, so if we cut down the fat in our diet, we put less on deposit. Aerobic exercise burns fat because, when we get mildly out of breath, the increased oxygen that we breathe in calls upon the fat in our muscles as well as our carbohydrate stores to provide energy. That's why marathon runners are so thin! Muscle-toning exercises are different, in that they work specific muscles, making them bigger and stronger. The bigger our muscles the higher our metabolic rate – that's the rate we burn off food.

You may be wondering if you will have enough willpower to see this programme through for the whole 28 days. It is quite a commitment and I can understand anyone having misgivings. There is absolutely no doubt that you can do it if you want to do it badly enough. This also applies to everything else in your life. Perhaps now would be a good time to recognise other ambitions you may have. Why not start thinking of all the things you would like to accomplish after you have achieved your new figure? Start a list of ambitions.

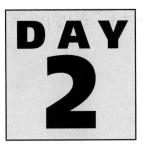

DAY 2

You know that you can succeed on this diet and exercise programme. As you approach Day 2, I hope you are feeling very positive about your chances of success. You should be feeling slimmer this morning, and this should encourage you to carry on for another day. Did you remember to pull your tummy in and stand tall at all times yesterday? It is worth persevering with this very good posture habit. Have a good day.

— Menu —

BREAKFAST

25g (1oz) PORRIDGE (see recipe, page 180)

OR

4 pieces of fresh fruit (e.g. 1 apple, 2 pears and a banana)

LUNCH

4 slices of light bread (max 200kcals) spread with reduced-oil salad dressing and made into sandwiches with lots of lettuce, tomatoes and cucumber, plus 1 × 150g (5oz) diet yogurt, any flavour

OR

1 cup of slimmer's cup-a-soup, plus 50g (2oz) chicken (with skin removed) or lean ham, served with a large salad, 115g (4oz) potatoes and a little reduced-oil salad dressing

DINNER

175g (6oz) white fish (cooked without fat) and unlimited vegetables. Serve with tomato sauce if desired
PLUS
115g (4oz) strawberries or similar plus 50g (2oz) diet yogurt

OR

BLACKEYE BEAN CASSEROLE
(see recipe, page 174) served with unlimited vegetables
PLUS
75g (3oz) low-fat fromage frais or 1 × 150g (5oz) diet yogurt

WARM UP – MOBILITY

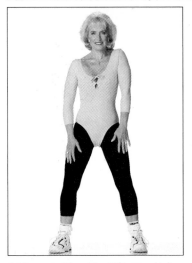

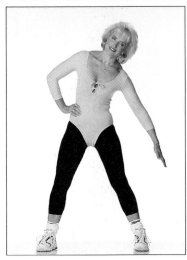

1 Alternate Shoulder Lifts Stand tall with feet apart, head up and shoulders back. Now lift alternate shoulders up and down. Do 12, changing sides each time.

2 Side Bends With feet apart and knees slightly bent, gently lean gently to one side, keeping the hips still and reaching out with one arm. Lift up and do the same to the other side. Repeat 6 times to each side.

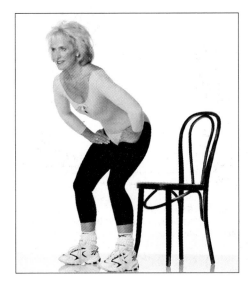

3 Knee Bends With legs wider than shoulder-width apart and feet turned out slightly, bend your knees in line with the toes, taking your hips back as if you were trying to sit in a chair. Come up without locking the knees fully. Repeat 6 times slowly.

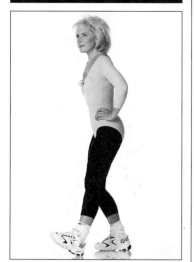

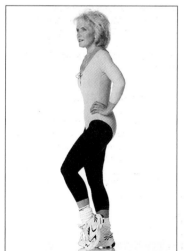

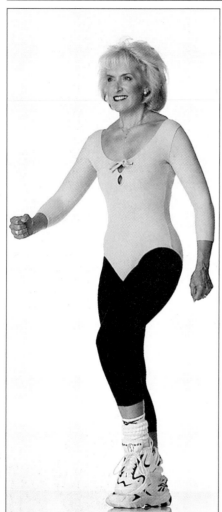

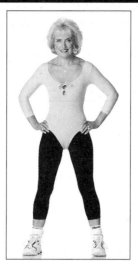

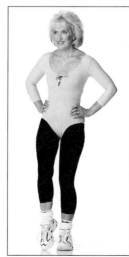

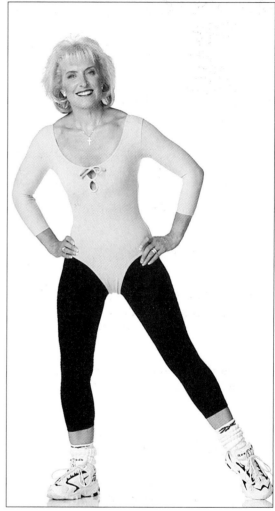

4 Heel/Toe Standing tall, with feet together, take your right heel diagonally out in front on the floor and then change to the toe. Keep alternating heel/toe 4 times altogether before changing to the left leg. The supporting knee should be slightly bent. Repeat again on each side.

5 March on the Spot Standing tall, with head up and shoulders back, march on the spot, allowing your arms to swing naturally. Make sure the heels land on the floor each time. March for 2 minutes.

6 Step Touch Take a step out to the right and bring the left toe to the right foot, then immediately step back to the left. Keep stepping from side to side rhythmically, bending your knees as the feet come together. Take 32 steps.

7 Weight Transfer Step out to the right, taking your weight on to the right foot and tapping the left toe to the floor with legs apart. Now transfer the weight to the left leg, tapping the right toe to the floor. Keep transferring your weight from one side to the other for 32 counts.

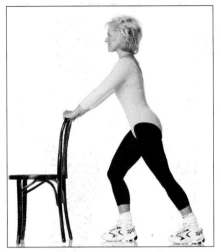

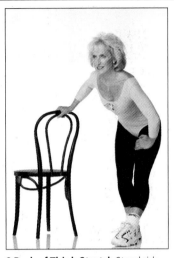

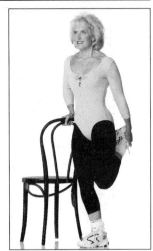

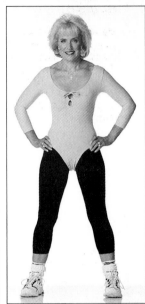

SEQUENCE 1

13a Step Touch Stand tall, with your hands on hips, and take a step out to the side with the right foot. Now tap the left foot close to the right foot and immediately step to the left, tapping the right foot to the left. Keep changing sides, bending your knees as the feet come together. Perform 8 times, then change to 13b.

8 Calf Stretch Hold on to the back of a chair and place one foot in front of the other, with the front leg bent and the back leg straight. Lean towards the front leg slightly and check that both feet point forward. Hold for 6 seconds, then change legs and repeat.

9 Back of Thigh Stretch Stand side-on to a chair and hold on to it for support. Bend the leg nearest to the chair and keep the other leg straight, with your hand on the thigh. Now lean forward, keeping your head in line and your back straight, until you feel a stretch in the back of the thigh. Hold for 6 seconds, then turn around to change legs and repeat.

10 Front of Thigh Stretch Still standing side-on to the chair, take hold of the outside leg around the ankle and bend the supporting knee slightly. Keep the knees together and push the outside hip forward to feel a stretch down the front of the thigh. Hold for 6 seconds, then turn around to change legs, and repeat.

11 Chest Stretch Sit upright on the edge of the chair, with feet flat on the floor. Take your hands behind you to hold the back of the chair, and feel a stretch across the chest. Hold for 6 seconds.

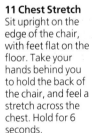

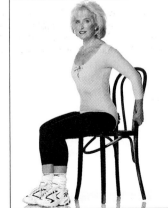

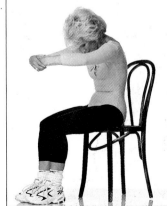

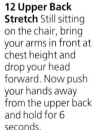

12 Upper Back Stretch Still sitting on the chair, bring your arms in front at chest height and drop your head forward. Now push your hands away from the upper back and hold for 6 seconds.

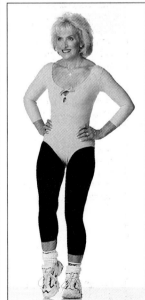

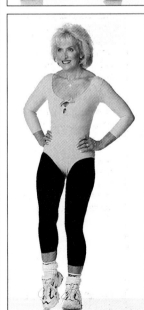

13b Double Side Steps Now take 2 steps out to the right and then back to the left. Make sure the whole foot makes contact with the floor and keep your tummy in and your back straight. Perform twice through and then go back to the single step touch.

Repeat this sequence 4 times.

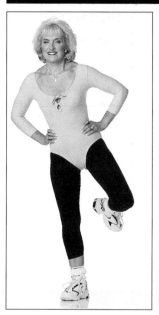

SEQUENCE 2

14a Hopscotch Take a step out to the right and bend your left heel up behind you, then step out to the left, bringing the right heel up. Repeat 8 times, then change to 14b.

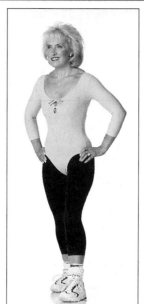
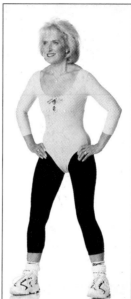
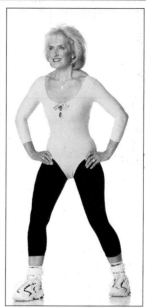
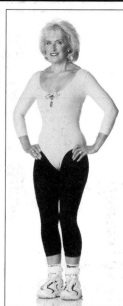

14b Walk Forward and Back
Step forward on the right leg and continue moving forward for 3 steps, and on the 4th count bring the left foot to tap to the right foot and clap your hands. Now step back with the left foot for 3 steps and on the 4th count bring the right foot to tap to the left foot and clap your hands. Repeat twice through before going back to 14a.

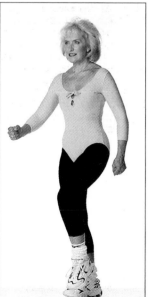

Repeat this sequence 4 times.

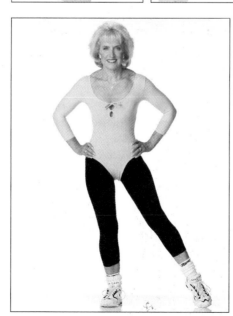

SEQUENCE 3

▲ **15a Box Step** This exercise has 4 counts. Take a step forward on the right foot, as if to the top right corner of a box (count 1). Now bring the left foot out to the top left corner (count 2). Step back again with the right (count 3) and follow with the left (count 4). Complete 4 full box steps before changing to 15b.

◀ **15b Half Jacks** Now tap the ball of the right foot out to the side. Bring the feet together and tap the left foot out. Keep changing sides, making sure you keep the knee of the supporting leg slightly bent and stand tall throughout. Repeat 8 times before going back to 15a.

Repeat this sequence 4 times.

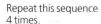

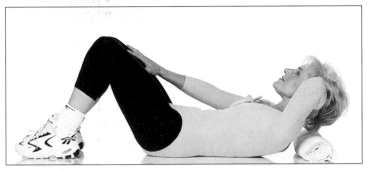

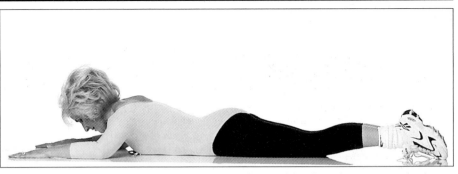

16 Easy Curl Lie on your back, with knees bent, feet flat on the floor, and your head resting on a rolled-up towel. Adopt the pelvic tilt position by pulling in your tummy and flattening it against the spine. With your left hand behind your head and the other hand resting on the right leg, gently lift your head and shoulders off the floor, keeping your chin off your chest, then lower again. Perform 4 times, breathing out as you lift and breathing in as you lower. Rest and repeat.

17 Back Raises Lie on your tummy, with your arms out in front and the elbows bent. Now gently raise your upper body from the floor, keeping the whole of the forearms on the floor. Look down at the floor all the time so that the neck stays long. Repeat 4 times, then rest and repeat.

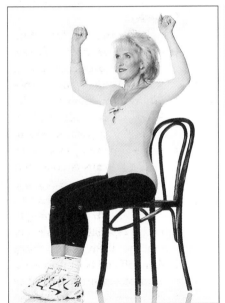

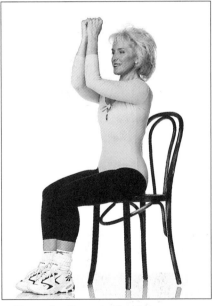

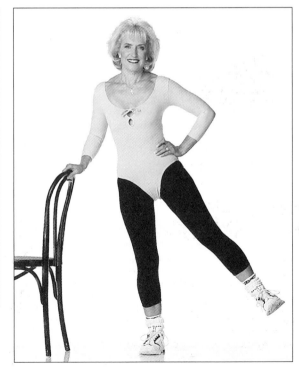

19 Standing Outer Thigh Lift Standing side-on to a chair, place one hand on the chair for support and the other hand on your hip. Keep the body upright and, with the leg nearest the chair slightly bent, lift the outside leg off the floor without leaning towards the chair. Lower again, then lift and lower 8 times before turning around to change legs and repeat.

18 Chest Toner Sitting towards the edge of a chair, with your feet flat on the floor, bring your arms out to the sides so that each arm forms a 90-degree angle at chest height. Now squeeze the elbows towards each other, keeping them in line with the chest. Breathe out as you bring them in, and breathe in as you open them again. Perform slowly and smoothly 6 times, then rest and repeat.

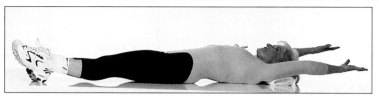

20 Full Body Stretch Lie on your back and take both arms overhead, stretching the legs away from you at the same time. Reach the arms as far away from the legs as is comfortable. Hold for 6 seconds, then release.

▶ **21 Spine Stretch** Come up into a box shape on hands and knees. Now pull your tummy in tightly, arching your back and tucking your hips under. Breathe normally. Hold for 8 seconds, then release.

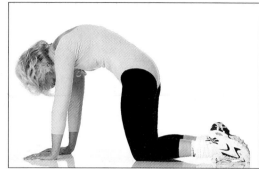

22 Chest Stretch Sitting cross-legged, with your back straight and your head up, take both hands behind you on the floor and pull your shoulder blades together at the back to feel a stretch across the chest. Hold for 8 seconds.

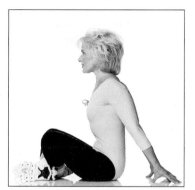

23 Outer Thigh Stretch Sit upright, with both legs out in front. Now take your bent right leg across the left knee, using the left hand to press it further across the body and placing the other hand on the floor for support. Hold for 8 seconds, then change legs and repeat.

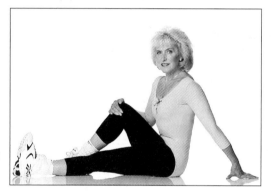

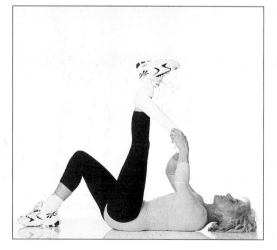

24 Front of Thigh Stretch Lie on your front, with your hands resting under your chin. Now, using your right hand, take hold of the right ankle (you can use a towel to assist if you find this difficult). Bring the heel close to the hip and push the hip down gently into the floor. Hold for 10 seconds, then change legs and repeat.

25 Back of Thigh Stretch Lie on your back, with knees bent and feet flat on the floor. Now take hold behind one leg, using a towel to assist, and ease the leg towards the chest. Try to keep the leg as straight as possible, with both hips remaining on the floor, to feel a stretch at the back of the thigh. Hold for 10 seconds, then change legs and repeat.

POSITIVE THOUGHT FOR THE DAY

Your body is beginning to become familiar with the various movements you are undertaking and will become fitter as each day passes. Your heart and lungs will benefit from the aerobic exercises, and your muscles will be challenged by the muscle-toning exercises. Perseverance and patience is the key to your success. These moves have been thoughtfully designed to give you maximum benefits and optimum results.

Soon you will look slimmer and younger and will walk with more confidence because the exercises will improve your posture. You should also be feeling more positive about yourself and your chances of success. I am sure you are going to receive many compliments because your appearance will improve tremendously. It isn't always easy to receive compliments, especially if you're not used to them. Don't shrug them off and be embarrassed, but accept them in the way they are intended – with grace and

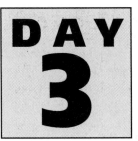

DAY 3

Two days of dieting completed and you've found muscles in your body you didn't know were there. Things are happening – your fat stores are depleting, your body is looking better already and you should be feeling more energetic. Now it's Day 3 and you can have a treat. It can be an extra glass of wine, an extra yogurt or a couple of pieces of fresh fruit – even a few sweets. However, if you don't want to eat or drink it today, save it up for another occasion.

Give your body a rest from the exercise programme today, but do try to be as active as possible in your daily activities. These regular 'rest days' help your muscles recover and your energy stores replenish.

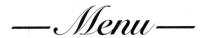

—Menu—

BREAKFAST

2 Weetabix (or 1 Weetabix plus a sliced banana) served with milk from allowance and 2 teaspoons sugar

OR

6 prunes soaked overnight in hot tea (ordinary or herbal tea is suitable)
and served with 1 × 150g (5oz) diet yogurt

LUNCH

RICE SALAD
(see recipe, page 182), plus 1 × 150g (5oz) diet yogurt

OR

5 Ryvitas spread with 115g (4oz) tuna (in brine) topped with sliced tomatoes, plus 1 piece of fresh fruit

DINNER

115g (4oz) lean steak or 175g (6oz) chicken (no skin) dry-fried or grilled, served with unlimited vegetables
PLUS
1 meringue basket filled with 50g (2oz) fresh fruit and topped with 50g (2oz) diet yogurt

OR

VEGETABLE BAKE
(see recipe, page 184)
PLUS
Stuffed apple: 1 apple, cored and filled with 25g (1oz) sultanas and artificial sweetener (if desired)
topped with 1 × 150g (5oz) diet yogurt

POSITIVE THOUGHT FOR THE DAY

It is a known fact that most people who attempt a new diet or exercise regime fail on Day 3. The very fact that you have reached this point means that you have crossed that most difficult threshold. Congratulations!

I would like you to become more aware of your own achievement and attributes from now on. Don't be self-critical. You have already proved to yourself that you can find enough willpower to stick to this programme for 3 days. I would like you to get to know your body better by looking in the mirror and seeing the improvements in your shape as each day goes by. Learn to recognise which areas are toning up and which are reducing. If you are dieting and exercising with a friend, make a point of noticing their progress too. From now on, it should get easier and the results should be even more rewarding. You'll be amazed how quickly you can see the results. You are probably finding yourself sleeping better too.

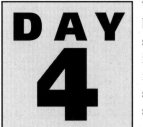

DAY 4

You are now at the halfway mark of the first week of this programme. Your body will be showing a significant improvement in posture and you should be feeling healthier. Soon you will be able to see your skin texture improving, and your new positive attitude towards yourself will give you a more sunny view on life in general. Try on your measuring garment and see if it has slackened off. Don't be tempted to wear it. It should be kept solely for the purpose of measuring.

Select from today's menu and enjoy the exercises which are specifically designed to work your body a little harder each day, giving it increased fitness and strength. Do only what you can and if the repetitions seem too challenging, then just do as many as are within your capability.

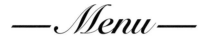

— Menu —

BREAKFAST

175g (6oz) fresh fruit salad topped with 1 × 150g (5oz) diet yogurt

OR

2 slices (50g/2oz) toast spread with Marmite and 50g (2oz) low-fat cottage cheese

LUNCH

50g (2oz) wholemeal bread spread with mustard and/or Branston pickle and made into open sandwiches with 50g (2oz) wafer thin ham, chicken or turkey and topped with sliced tomatoes

OR

Jacket potato (approx. 175g/6oz) topped with 25g (1oz) sweetcorn and 75g (3oz) low-fat cottage cheese

DINNER

CHICKEN CHOP SUEY (see recipe, page 000)
PLUS
1 × 150g (5oz) diet yogurt

OR

VEGETARIAN CHOP SUEY
Cook as recipe for CHICKEN CHOP SUEY (see page 175), excluding the chicken, and serve with unlimited boiled brown rice and soy sauce
PLUS
1 low-fat fromage frais or 1 × 150g (5oz) diet yogurt

WARM UP – MOBILITY

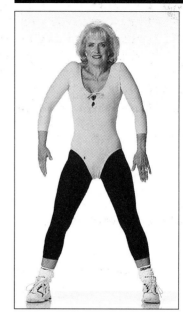

1 Double Shoulder Lifts
Standing with feet apart, shoulders back and head up, smoothly raise both shoulders up towards the ears, then press them down again. Perform 8 times under control.

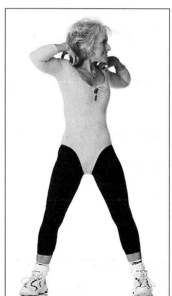

2 Waist Twists
Stand upright, with feet apart, tummy pulled in and knees slightly bent. Now place your hands on your shoulders and twist round as far as you can go, keeping the hips facing forward. Return to face front and do the same to the other side. Keep it smooth and controlled. Do 12, changing sides each time.

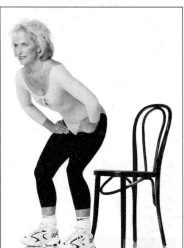

3 Knee Bends
With legs wider than shoulder-width apart and feet turned out slightly, bend your knees in line with the toes, taking your hips back as if you were trying to sit in a chair. Come up without locking the knees fully. Repeat 6 times slowly.

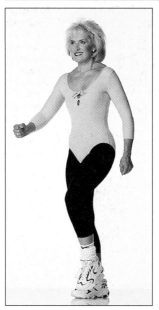

◀ **5 March on the Spot**
Standing tall, with head up and shoulders back, march on the spot, allowing your arms to swing naturally. Make sure the heels land on the floor each time. March for 2 minutes.

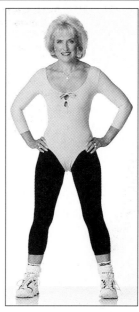

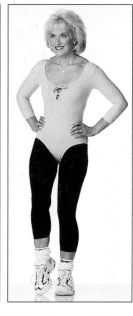

▶ **6 Double Side Steps**
Take 2 steps out to the right and then back to the left. Make sure the whole foot makes contact with the floor and keep your tummy in and your back straight. Repeat to both sides 4 times altogether.

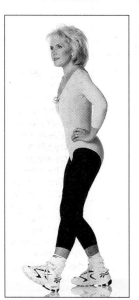

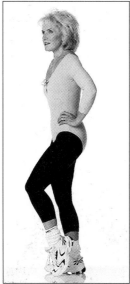

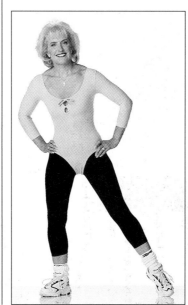

7 Weight Transfer
Step out to the right, taking your weight on to the right foot and tapping the left toe to the floor with legs apart. Now transfer the weight to the left leg, tapping the right toe to the floor. Keep transferring your weight from one side to the other for 32 counts.

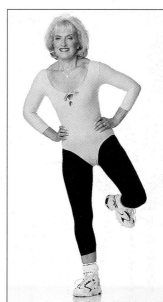

8 Hopscotch Take a step out to the right and bend your left heel up behind you, then step out to the left, bringing the right heel up. Repeat 8 times.

4 Heel/Toe Standing tall, with feet together, take your right heel diagonally out in front on the floor and then change to the toe. Keep alternating heel/toe 4 times altogether before changing to the left leg. The supporting knee should be slightly bent. Repeat again on each side.

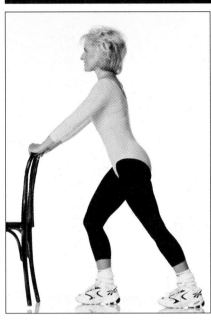

9 Calf Stretch
Hold on to the back of a chair and place one foot in front of the other, with the front leg bent and the back leg straight. Lean towards the front leg slightly and check that both feet point forward. Hold for 6 seconds, then change legs and repeat.

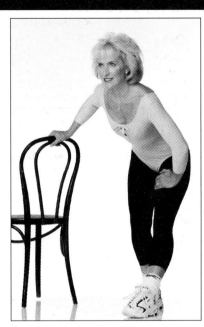

10 Back of Thigh Stretch
Stand side-on to a chair and hold on to it for support. Bend the leg nearest to the chair and keep the other leg straight, with your hand on the thigh. Now lean forward, keeping your head in line and your back straight, until you feel a stretch in the back of the thigh. Hold for 6 seconds, then turn around to change legs and repeat.

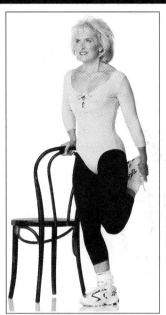

11 Front of Thigh Stretch
Still standing side-on to the chair, take hold of the outside leg around the ankle and bend the supporting knee slightly. Keep the knees together and push the outside hip forward to feel a stretch down the front of the thigh. Hold for 6 seconds, then turn around to change legs, and repeat.

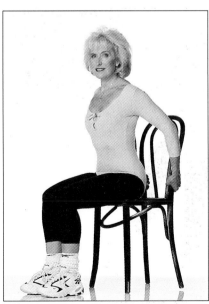

◀ **12 Chest Stretch** Sit upright on the edge of the chair, with feet flat on the floor. Take your hands behind you to hold the back of the chair, and feel a stretch across the chest. Hold for 6 seconds.

▶ **13 Upper Back Stretch** Still sitting on the chair, bring your arms in front at chest height and drop your head forward. Now push your hands away from the upper back and hold for 6 seconds.

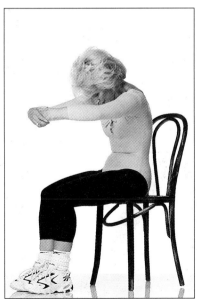

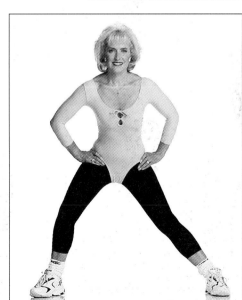

14 Inner Thigh Stretch
Standing with feet wide apart, turn one foot out slightly and bend the knee in line with the foot. Keep the other leg straight, with the foot pointing forward, and feel the stretch on the inside of the straight leg. Hold for 6 seconds, then change legs and repeat.

SEQUENCE 1

15a Step Touch
Stand tall, with your hands on hips, and take a step out to the side with the right foot. Now tap the left foot close to the right foot and immediately step to the left, tapping the right foot to the left. Keep changing sides, bending your knees as the feet come together. Perform 8 times, then change to 15b.

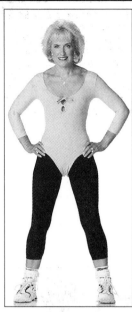

15b Double Side Steps Now take 2 steps out to the right and then back to the left. Make sure the whole foot makes contact with the floor and keep your tummy in and your back straight. Perform twice through and then go back to the single step touch.

Repeat this sequence 5 times.

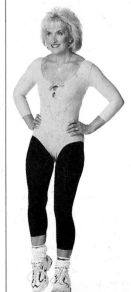
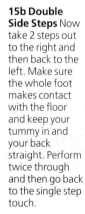

SEQUENCE 2

16a Hopscotch
Take a step out to the right and bend your left heel up behind you, then step out to the left, bringing the right heel up. Repeat 8 times, then change to 16b.

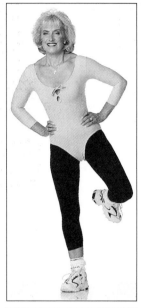

16b Walk Forward and Back Step forward on the right leg and continue moving forward for 3 steps, and on the 4th count bring the left foot to tap to the right foot and clap your hands. Now step back with the left foot for 3 steps and on the 4th count bring the right foot to tap to the left foot and clap your hands. Repeat twice through before going back to 16a.

Repeat this sequence 5 times.

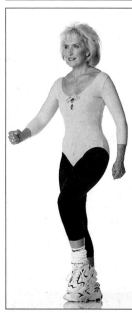
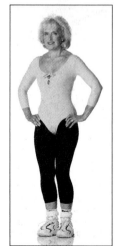

SEQUENCE 3

17a Box Step This exercise has 4 counts. Take a step forward on the right foot, as if to the top right corner of a box (count 1). Now bring the left foot out to the top left corner (count 2). Step back again with the right (count 3) and follow with the left (count 4). Complete 4 full box steps before changing to 17b.

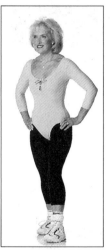
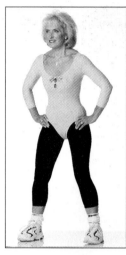
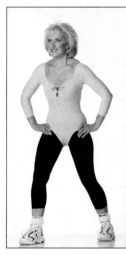

17b Half Jacks
Now tap the ball of the right foot out to the side. Bring the feet together and tap the left foot out. Keep changing sides, making sure you keep the knee of the supporting leg slightly bent and stand tall throughout. Repeat 8 times before going back to 17a.

Repeat this sequence 4 times.

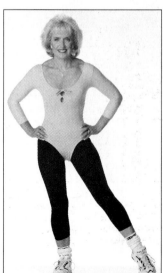

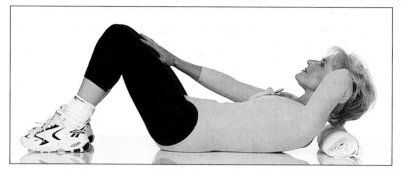

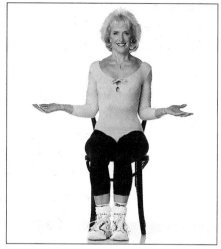

19 Posture Squeezes Sit upright on a chair, with your feet flat on the floor, and place your elbows close to your waist, with your forearms out in front and your palms facing up, as if you were holding a tray. Now gently take your forearms out to the sides as shown to feel your shoulder blades squeeze closer together at the back. Hold momentarily, then release. Keep it slow and smooth. Do 4, then rest and repeat.

18 Easy Curl Lie on your back, with knees bent, feet flat on the floor, and your head resting on a rolled-up towel. Adopt the pelvic tilt position by pulling in your tummy and flattening it against the spine. With your left hand behind your head and the other hand resting on the right leg, gently lift your head and shoulders off the floor, keeping your chin off your chest, then lower again. Perform 4 times, breathing out as you lift and breathing in as you lower. Rest and repeat.

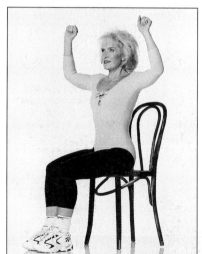

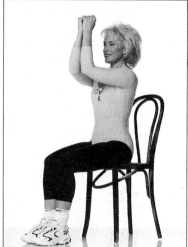

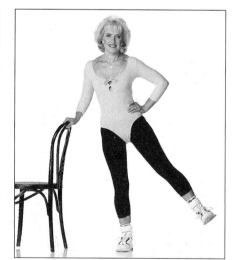

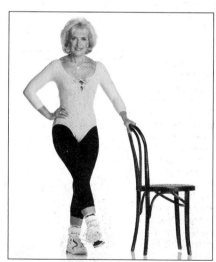

20 Chest Toner Sitting towards the edge of a chair, with your feet flat on the floor, bring your arms out to the sides so that each arm forms a 90-degree angle at chest height. Now squeeze the elbows towards each other, keeping them in line with the chest. Breathe out as you bring them in, and breathe in as you open them again. Perform slowly and smoothly 6 times, then rest and repeat.

21 Standing Outer Thigh Lift Standing side-on to a chair, place one hand on the chair for support and other hand on your hip. Keep the body upright and, with the leg nearest the chair slightly bent, lift the outside leg off the floor without leaning towards the chair. Lower again, then lift and lower 8 times before turning around to change legs and repeat.

22 Standing Inner Thigh Toner Still standing side-on to the chair, take your weight on to the inside leg. Now, keeping the body upright, draw the outside leg up and across the front of the body, then lower it again. The supporting leg should stay soft. Repeat 8 times, lifting and lowering under control. Turn around to repeat on the other leg.

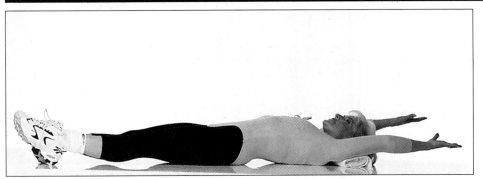

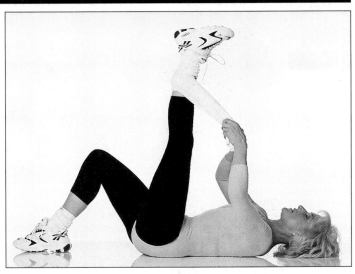

23 Full Body Stretch Lie on your back and take both arms overhead, stretching the legs away from you at the same time. Reach the arms as far away from the legs as is comfortable. Hold for 6 seconds, then release.

▶ **24 Back of Thigh Stretch** Lie on your back, with knees bent and feet flat on the floor. Now take hold behind one leg, using a towel to assist, and ease the leg towards the chest. Try to keep the leg as straight as possible, with both hips remaining on the floor, to feel a stretch at the back of the thigh. Hold for 10 seconds, then change legs and repeat.

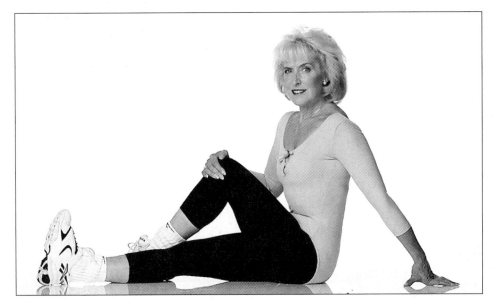

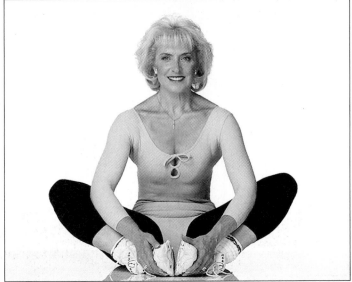

25 Outer Thigh Stretch Sit upright, with both legs out in front. Now take your bent right leg across the left knee, using the left hand to press it further across the body and placing the other hand on the floor for support. Hold for 8 seconds, then change legs and repeat.

26 Inner Thigh Stretch Sit with the soles of the feet together and hold your ankles with your hands. Try to place the elbows on the inside of the knees and press down gently to encourage them further towards the floor, and feel the stretch in the inner thigh area. Hold for 10 seconds.

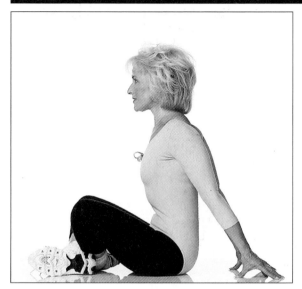

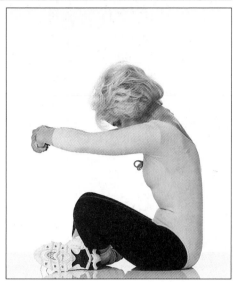

27 Chest Stretch Sitting cross-legged, with your back straight and your head up, take both hands behind you on the floor and pull your shoulder blades together at the back to feel a stretch across the chest. Hold for 8 seconds.

28 Upper Back Stretch Still sitting cross-legged on the floor, bring your arms forward at chest height. Gently lower your head and press your arms further away from the upper back to feel the stretch across your shoulders. Hold for 8 seconds.

POSITIVE THOUGHT FOR THE DAY

You must be delighted with your progress, and I hope this feeling of wellbeing will encourage you to continue with the programme. I am sure that you will be feeling more confident not only about your appearance, but also about your ability to persevere. Often in life we are prevented from realising our true potential because we feel restricted, or are harbouring some feelings that we would love to share.

It may be that we have upset someone and a rift exists. We dread facing them because we are frightened of what the other people might say. Often such matters are trivial, yet they can have an immeasurably detrimental effect on our lives. If you have anything that is troubling you today, I strongly recommend that you face it head-on. Pick up the phone and speak to the person concerned. If they have upset you, perhaps they are hoping you will make the first move. If you can clear up this problem, you can look forward to a happier future.

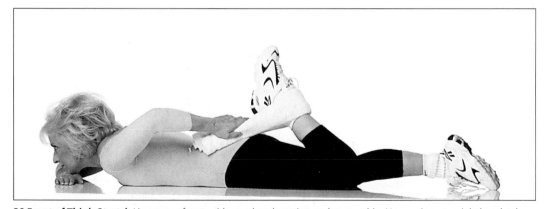

29 Front of Thigh Stretch Lie on your front, with your hands resting under your chin. Now, using your right hand, take hold of the right ankle (you can use a towel to assist if you find this difficult). Bring the heel close to the hip and push the hip down gently into the floor. Hold for 10 seconds, then change legs and repeat.

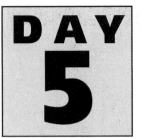

DAY 5

Did you look slimmer this morning when you looked at yourself sideways in the mirror? Try to assess your progress daily in this way. Weighing scales are fine as a guide once a week, but because our fluid levels change from day to day according to what we eat or drink, they sometimes give a misleading reading. Also, the menstrual cycles of women can seriously disrupt fluid levels, causing increases of several pounds in some cases. I invariably gain weight if I've eaten rice the evening before, because it retains water and is often served with spicy food which is dehydrating. So if you have a special occasion for which you want to feel particularly slim, don't eat rice the day before!

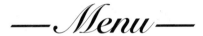

—Menu—

BREAKFAST

½ a fresh grapefruit plus 1 small egg, poached or boiled,
served with 25g (1oz) wholemeal toast

OR

50g (2oz) Kellogg's All-Bran served with milk from allowance and 1 teaspoon of sugar

LUNCH

1 × 200g (7oz) tin of baked beans eaten cold, plus 2 pieces of fresh fruit
and 1 × 150g (5oz) diet yogurt

OR

1 × 50g (2oz) bread roll spread with reduced-oil salad dressing and filled with salad,
25g (1oz) wafer thin ham or chicken, plus 1 banana

DINNER

SHEPHERD'S PIE (see recipe, page 182)
PLUS
PEARS IN MERINGUE (see recipe, page 180)

OR

VEGETARIAN SHEPHERD'S PIE (see recipe, page 185)
PLUS
1 × 150g (5oz) diet yogurt

WARM UP – MOBILITY

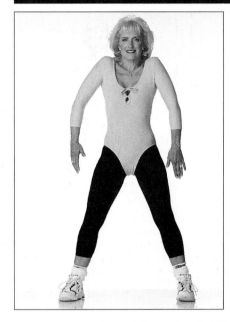

1 Double Shoulder Lifts Standing with feet apart, shoulders back and head up, smoothly raise both shoulders up towards the ears then press them down again. Perform 8 times under control.

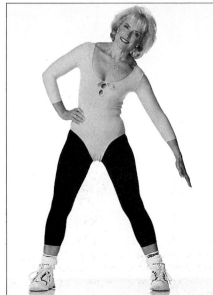

2 Side Bends With feet apart and knees slightly bent, gently lean to one side, keeping the hips still and reaching out with one arm. Lift up and do the same to the other side. Repeat 6 times to each side.

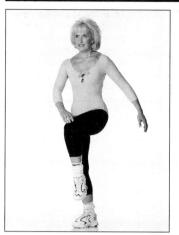

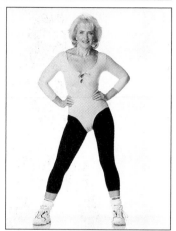

3 Knee Lifts Take a step out to the side with the right leg then lift the left knee up to waist height, keeping your back straight and your head up. Try to touch the raised knee with the opposite hand. Perform 24, alternating legs.

4 Hip Shifts Stand with feet wide apart and knees slightly bent. Now lift alternate hips, keeping both heels on the floor. Keep the movement slow and controlled. Do 12, changing sides each time.

6 Double Side Steps
Take 2 steps out to the right and then back to the left. Make sure the whole foot makes contact with the floor and keep your tummy in and your back straight. Repeat 4 times to each side.

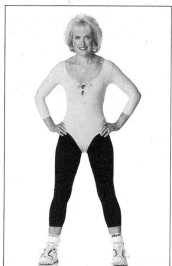

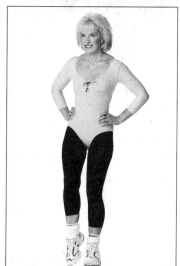

7 Weight Transfer Step out to the right, taking your weight on to the right foot and tapping the left toe to the floor with legs apart. Now transfer the weight to the left leg, tapping the right toe to the floor. Keep transferring your weight from one side to the other for 32 counts.

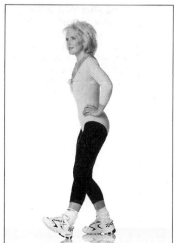

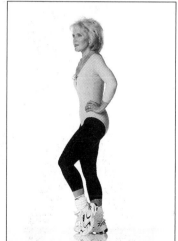

5 Heel/Toe Standing tall, with feet together, take your right heel diagonally out in front on the floor and then change to the toe. Keep alternating heel/toe 4 times altogether before changing to the left leg. The supporting knee should be slightly bent. Repeat again on each side.

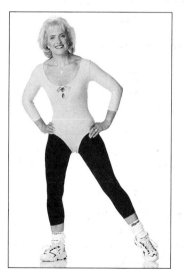

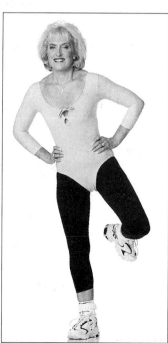

▶ **8 Hopscotch** Take a step out to the right and bend your left heel up behind you, then step out to the left, bringing the right heel up. Repeat 8 times.

9 Calf Stretch Hold on to the back of a chair and place one foot in front of the other, with the front leg bent and the back leg straight. Lean towards the front leg slightly and check that both feet point forward. Hold for 6 seconds, then change legs and repeat.

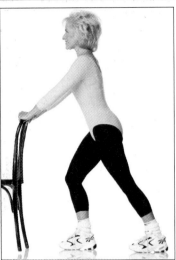

10 Back of Thigh Stretch Stand side-on to the chair and hold on to it for support. Bend the leg nearest to the chair and keep the other leg straight, with your hand on the thigh. Now lean forward, keeping your head in line and your back straight, until you feel a stretch in the back of the thigh. Hold for 6 seconds, then turn around to change legs and repeat.

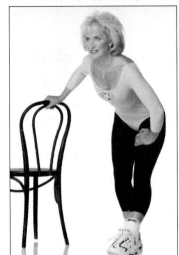

▼ **11 Front of Thigh Stretch** Still standing side-on to the chair, take hold of the outside leg around the ankle and bend the supporting knee slightly. Keep the knees together and push the outside hip forward to feel a stretch down the front of the thigh. Hold for 6 seconds, then turn around to change legs, and repeat.

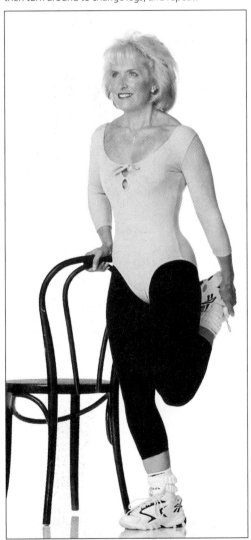

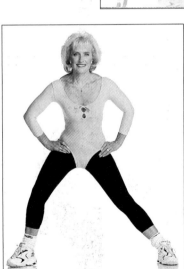

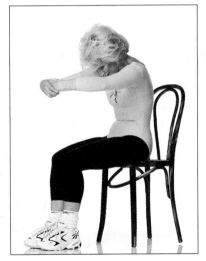

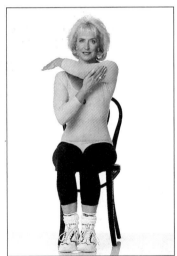

12 Inner Thigh Stretch Standing with feet wide apart, turn one foot out slightly and bend the knee in line with the foot. Keep the other leg straight, with the foot pointing forward, and feel the stretch on the inside of the straight leg. Hold for 6 seconds, then change legs and repeat.

13 Upper Back Stretch Sit upright on the edge of a chair. Bring your arms in front at chest height and drop your head forward. Now push your hands away from the upper back and hold for 6 seconds.

14 Easy Tricep Stretch Still sitting upright on the chair, bring one arm across the chest and gently press at the back of the arm with the other hand to push the arm back further. Hold for 6 seconds, then change arms and repeat.

Some easy arm movements are introduced today, but leave them out if you prefer.

SEQUENCE 1

15a Step Touch with Elbow Curls Step to alternate sides, bending your knees as the feet come together. At the same time, bend alternate elbows, keeping them close to the waist. Perform rhythmically 8 times before changing to 15b.

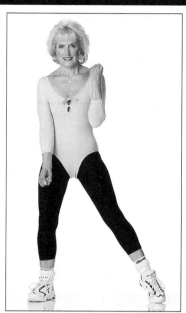

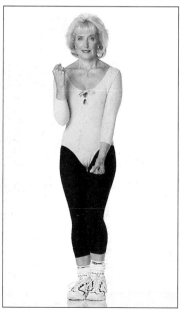

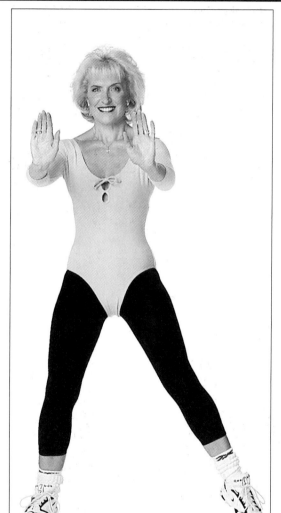

15b Double Steps with Chest Press Take 2 steps to the side, pressing the arms in front at the same time. Repeat twice to each side before going back to 15a.

Repeat this sequence 5 times.

SEQUENCE 2

16a Hopscotch Take a step out to the side and bend one knee up behind you, lifting the heel towards the hip. Step wider now and bend your knees more. Repeat 8 times, changing legs each time, before moving on to 16b.

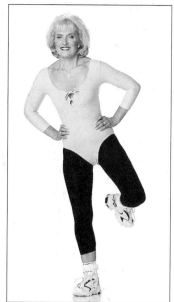

16b Walk Forward and Back Step forward on the right leg and continue moving forward for 3 steps, and on the 4th count bring the left foot to tap to the right foot and clap your hands. Now step back with the left foot for 3 steps and on the 4th count bring the right foot to tap to the left foot and clap your hands. Repeat twice through before going back to 16a.

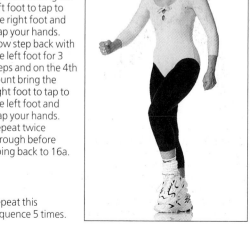

Repeat this sequence 5 times.

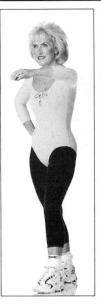
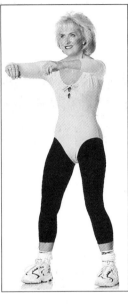
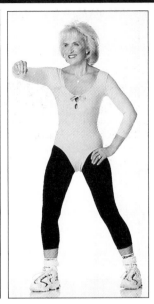
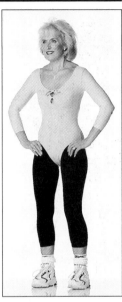

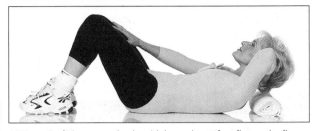

18 Easy Curl Lie on your back, with knees bent, feet flat on the floor, and your head resting on a rolled-up towel. Adopt the pelvic tilt position by pulling in your tummy and flattening it against the spine. With your left hand behind your head and the other hand resting on the right leg, gently lift your head and shoulders off the floor, keeping your chin off your chest, then lower again. Perform 4 times, breathing out as you lift and breathing in as you lower. Rest and repeat.

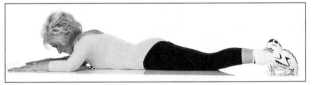

19 Back Raises Lie on your tummy, with your arms out in front and the elbows bent. Now gently raise your upper body from the floor, keeping the whole of the forearms on the floor. Look down at the floor all the time so that the neck stays long. Repeat 4 times, then rest and repeat.

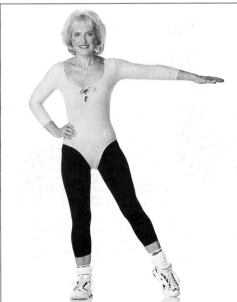

SEQUENCE 3

▲ **17a Box Step with Arms** As you step forward on the right foot, take the right arm forward at chest height, then follow with the left foot and arm. As you step back, bring each arm back to the hips. You should step wider and deeper now as you need to work harder. Complete 4 complete box steps before moving on to 17b.

◀ **17b Half Jacks with Single Arm** Now take the right toe to touch out at the side, pushing the arm out in the same direction. Bring the feet back together and push out to the other side. Bend the supporting leg more and move more strongly. Repeat 8 times to alternate sides before going back to 17a.

Repeat this sequence 5 times to complete your aerobics session.

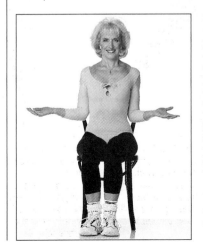

20 Posture Squeezes Sit upright on a chair, with your feet flat on the floor, and place your elbows close to your waist, with your forearms out in front and your palms facing up, as if you were holding a tray. Now gently take your forearms out to the sides as shown to feel your shoulder blades squeeze closer together at the back. Hold momentarily, then release. Keep it slow and smooth. Do 4, then rest and repeat.

21 Underarm Toner Still sitting on the chair, with feet flat on the floor and the trunk upright, take your elbows as far behind you as you can and lean forward slightly. Keep your elbows back as you extend your arms behind. Do 6 slowly, then rest and repeat.

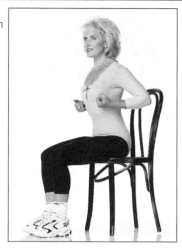 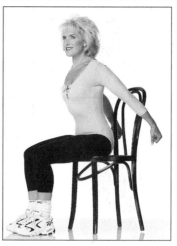

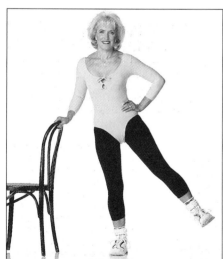

22 Standing Outer Thigh Lift Standing side-on to a chair, place one hand on the chair for support and other hand on your hip. Keep the body upright and, with the leg nearest the chair slightly bent, lift the outside leg off the floor without leaning towards the chair. Lower again, then lift and lower 8 times before turning around to change legs and repeat.

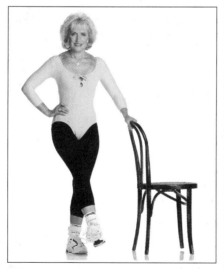

23 Standing Inner Thigh Toner Still standing side-on to the chair, take your weight on to the inside leg. Now, keeping the body upright, draw the outside leg up and across the front of the body, then lower it again. The supporting leg should stay soft. Repeat 8 times, lifting and lowering under control. Turn around to repeat on the other leg.

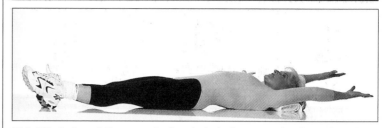

24 Full Body Stretch Lie on your back and take both arms overhead, stretching the legs away from you at the same time. Reach the arms as far away from the legs as is comfortable. Hold for 6 seconds then release.

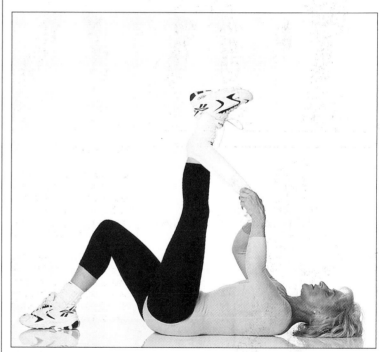

25 Back of Thigh Stretch Lie on your back, with knees bent and feet flat on the floor. Now take hold behind one leg, using a towel to assist, and ease the leg towards the chest. Try to keep the leg as straight as possible, with both hips remaining on the floor, to feel a stretch at the back of the thigh. Hold for 10 seconds, then change legs and repeat.

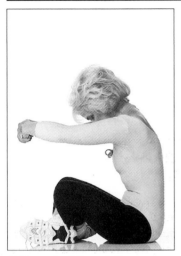

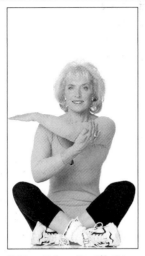

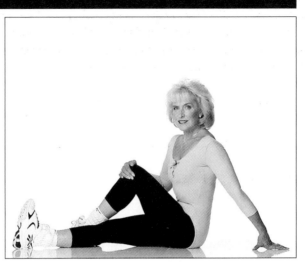

26 Upper Back Stretch Sit cross-legged on the floor and bring your arms forward at chest height. Gently lower your head and press your arms further away from the upper back to feel the stretch across your shoulders. Hold for 8 seconds.

27 Easy Tricep Stretch Bring one arm across in front of the chest. Place the other hand at the back of the upper arm and gently press further across to feel a stretch in the underarm area. Hold for 6 seconds, then change arms and repeat.

28 Outer Thigh Stretch Sit upright, with both legs out in front. Now take your bent right leg across the left knee, using the left hand to press it further across the body and placing the other hand on the floor for support. Hold for 8 seconds, then change legs and repeat.

29 Inner Thigh Stretch Sit with the soles of the feet together and hold your ankles with your hands. Try to place the elbows on the insides of the knees and press down gently to encourage them further towards the floor, and feel the stretch in the inner thigh area. Hold for 10 seconds.

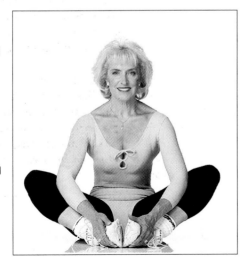

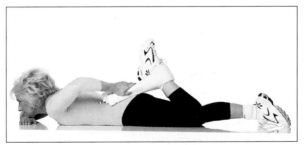

30 Front of Thigh Stretch Lie on your front, with your hands resting under your chin. Now, using your right hand, take hold of the right ankle (you can use a towel to assist if you find this difficult). Bring the heel close to the hip and push the hip down gently into the floor. Hold for 10 seconds, then change legs and repeat.

POSITIVE THOUGHT FOR THE DAY

If you prefer one day's menu to another, make a note of it and return to it in place of one that doesn't take your fancy. After all, the most successful diet will be the one that you enjoy. The important thing is that you don't feel hungry.

Today I would like you to think about taking up a new interest or hobby. Ideally, it should enable you to burn up a little more energy and help you to become fitter. The fitter we become and the more energy we expend on a regular basis, the easier it is for us to maintain our new figure. In making your selection, please eliminate from your vocabulary the words 'I can't'. How do you know you can't do something unless you try? I always suggest that people keep a note-book to list the long-term and short-term aims that they would like to achieve. So today please consider what you would like to achieve most. I have found that if you become happy with your body, you can actually accomplish a lot more in other ways. Now that you have made a very real commitment towards achieving your new shape, you will automatically gain self-esteem and extra energy.

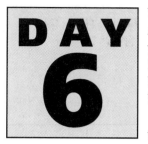
DAY 6

Yesterday I talked about having a more positive attitude towards yourself. As we near the end of this first week of body reshaping, I sincerely hope you are feeling better about yourself and more optimistic about the future. It won't be many days now before you see a real improvement in your basic shape. Try on your measuring garment. See how much looser it has become.

Today, you can have another rest day from the exercises, but remember to stay active.

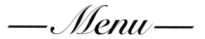

—Menu—

BREAKFAST

½ a melon, plus 1 × 150g (5oz) diet yogurt

OR

25g (1oz) very lean bacon or 2 turkey rashers well-grilled, served with 200g (7oz) tinned tomatoes and 15g (½oz) toast

LUNCH

1 × 200g (7oz) tin of spaghetti in tomato sauce served on 25g (1oz) toast, plus 1 piece of fresh fruit

OR

1 slimmer's cup-a-soup, plus 2 pieces of fresh fruit and 2 × 150g (2 × 5oz) diet yogurts

DINNER

PRAWN CURRY
(see recipe, page 181)
PLUS
PEARS IN RED WINE
(see recipe, page 180)

OR

VEGETABLE CURRY
(see recipe, page 184)
PLUS
115g (4oz) fresh fruit salad and 1 × 150g (5oz) diet yogurt

POSITIVE THOUGHT FOR THE DAY

Please continue to view your progress in the mirror and realise that it is only one more day before you measure and weigh yourself to enter your reduced (I hope!) statistics on the Weight and Inch Loss Record Chart.

Today, although you won't be doing the exercise programme, try to be as energetic as possible in all that you do, by putting a little extra effort into everything. Tomorrow is Day 7, and you will need to make a concerted effort to ensure that the results at the beginning of Day 8 really demonstrate your progress through the week. Plan to do something that will take you out of the house and, perhaps, go for a long walk.

Please try to be really strong tonight and don't cheat at all. You have done so well to get to this point, it is vital that you stay on the rails until the first weighing and measuring day. And remember that, if you do cheat, the only person you are letting down is yourself. It just isn't worth it.

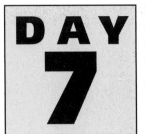

DAY 7

This is the last day of Week 1. If you've come this far you can be confident of reaching Day 28. The more you manage to re-educate your eating habits and energise your body, the more likely you are to continue in the long term. The exercises are becoming a little more challenging, but they are having an even greater benefit on your body. Be sure never to rush them, but feel how they are working and toning your muscles as never before.

Keep as busy as possible today and remember to hold yourself tall, and your tummy in. You will not only look much slimmer but you will feel it too. Think positively and try to make the most of your appearance so that you feel your absolute best all day. Enjoy your day and smile at the world.

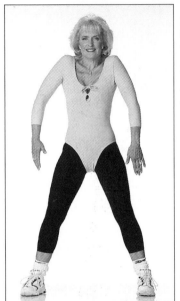

1 Double Shoulder Lifts
Standing with feet apart, shoulders back and head up, smoothly raise both shoulders up towards the ears then press them down again. Perform 8 times under control.

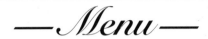

—Menu—

BREAKFAST

150g (5oz) diet yogurt mixed with 15g (½oz) oats, 15g (½oz) sultanas and 75g (3oz) sliced banana

OR

175g (6oz) tinned grapefruit in natural juice topped with a grapefruit yogurt

LUNCH

115g (4oz) roast lean meat or 175g (6oz) chicken (no skin) served with DRY-ROAST POTATOES (see recipe, page 176) and unlimited vegetables and gravy made with powder or low-fat granules

PLUS

ORANGES IN COINTREAU
(see recipe, page 179)

OR

VEGETARIAN GOULASH
(see recipe, page 185)

PLUS

115g (4oz) fresh fruit salad topped with 1 × 150g (5oz) diet yogurt

SUPPER

50g (2oz) wholemeal toast, topped with 200g (7oz) baked beans, plus 1 piece of fresh fruit

OR

50g (2oz) wholemeal bread spread with a mixture of 1 part tomato ketchup and 1 part reduced-oil salad dressing and made into sandwiches with lettuce and 15g (4oz) prawns, plus 1 × 150g (5oz) diet yogurt

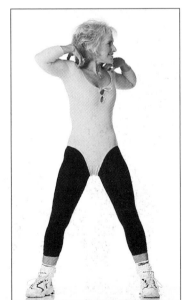

2 Waist Twists
Stand upright, with feet apart, tummy pulled in and knees slightly bent. Now place your hands on your shoulders and twist round as far as you can go, keeping the hips facing forward. Return to face front and do the same to the other side. Keep it smooth and controlled. Do 12, changing sides each time.

3 Knee Lifts
Take a step out to the side with the right leg then lift the left knee up to waist height, keeping your back straight and your head up. Try to touch the raised knee with the opposite hand. Perform 24, alternating legs.

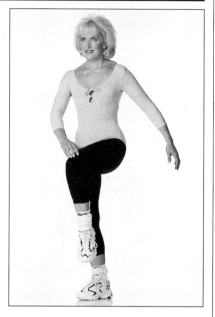

5 March on the Spot Standing tall, with head up and shoulders back, march on the spot, allowing your arms to swing naturally. Make sure the heels land on the floor each time. March for 2 minutes.

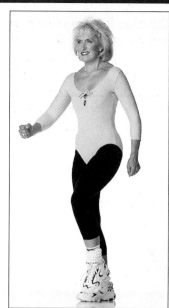

6 Weight Transfer Step out to the right, taking your weight on to the right foot and tapping the left toe to the floor with legs apart. Now transfer the weight to the left leg, tapping the right toe to the floor. Keep transferring your weight from one side to the other for 32 counts.

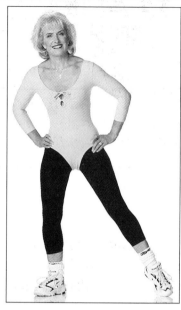

4 Knee Bends
With legs wider than shoulder-width apart and feet turned out slightly, bend your knees in line with the toes, taking your hips back as if you were trying to sit in a chair. Come up without locking the knees fully. Repeat 6 times slowly.

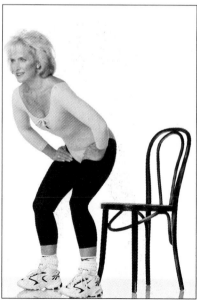

7 Double Side Steps Take 2 steps out to the right and then back to the left. Make sure the whole foot makes contact with the floor and keep your tummy in and your back straight. Repeat to both sides 4 times altogether.

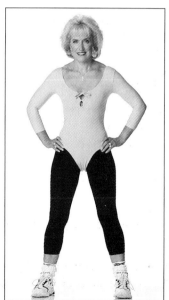

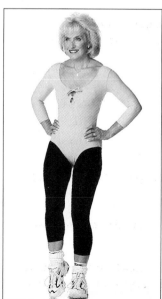

8 Calf Stretch
Hold on to the back of a chair and place one foot in front of the other, with the front leg bent and the back leg straight. Lean towards the front leg slightly and check that both feet point forward. Hold for 6 seconds, then change legs and repeat.

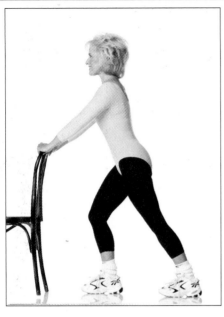

9 Back of Thigh Stretch Stand side-on to the chair and hold on to it for support. Bend the leg nearest to the chair and keep the other leg straight, with your hand on the thigh. Now lean forward, keeping your head in line and your back straight, until you feel a stretch in the back of the thigh. Hold for 6 seconds, then turn around to change legs and repeat.

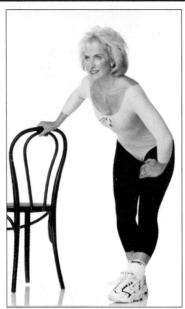

10 Front of Thigh Stretch
Still standing side-on to the chair, take hold of the outside leg around the ankle and bend the supporting knee slightly. Keep the knees together and push the outside hip forward to feel a stretch down the front of the thigh. Hold for 6 seconds, then turn around to change legs, and repeat.

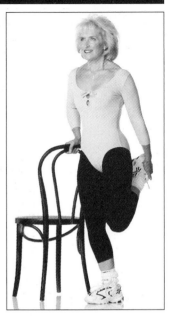

11 Inner Thigh Stretch
Standing with feet wide apart, turn one foot out slightly and bend the knee in line with the foot. Keep the other leg straight, with the foot pointing forward, and feel the stretch on the inside of the straight leg. Hold for 6 seconds, then change legs and repeat.

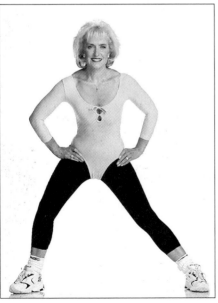

12 Chest Stretch Sit upright on the edge of a chair, with feet flat on the floor. Take your hands behind you to hold the back of the chair, and feel a stretch across the chest. Hold for 6 seconds.

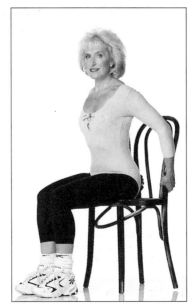

13 Easy Tricep Stretch Still sitting upright on the chair, bring one arm across the chest and gently press at the back of the arm with the other hand to push the arm back further. Hold for 6 seconds, then change arms and repeat.

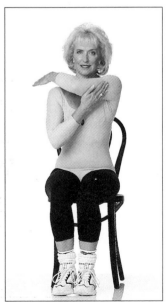

Try to add some more intensity to this session now by taking bigger steps and bending your knees more. This way, the exercise is far more effective.

SEQUENCE 1

14a Step Touch with Elbow Curls

Step to alternate sides, bending your knees as the feet come together. At the same time, bend alternate elbows, keeping them close to the waist. Perform rhythmically 8 times before changing to 14b.

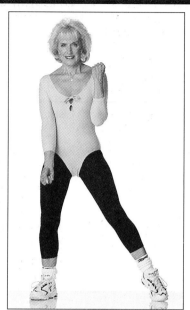

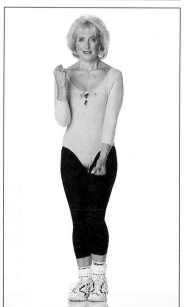

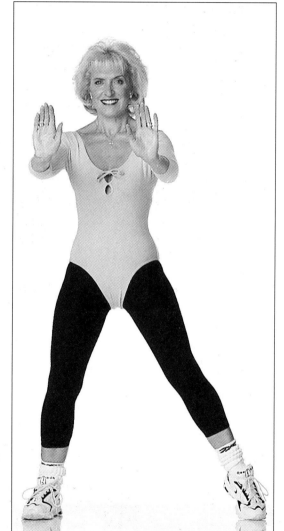

14b Double Steps with Chest Press Take 2 steps to the side, pressing the arms in front at the same time. Repeat twice to each side before going back to 14a.

Repeat this sequence 5 times.

SEQUENCE 2

15a Hopscotch

Take a step out to the side and bend one knee up behind you, lifting the heel toward the hip. Step wider now and bend your knees more. Repeat 8 times, changing legs each time, before moving on to 15b.

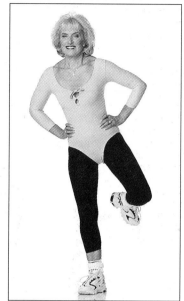

15b Walk Forward and Back Walk forward for 3 steps and on the 4th count tap the feet together and clap your hands. Now travel further on the walk and add more arm swing. Repeat forward and back twice before going back to 15a.

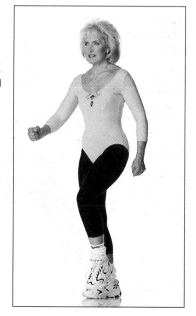

Repeat this sequence 5 times.

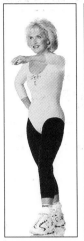
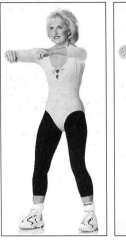
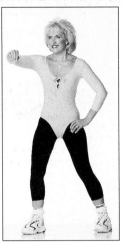
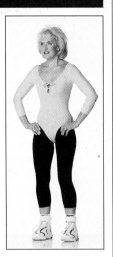

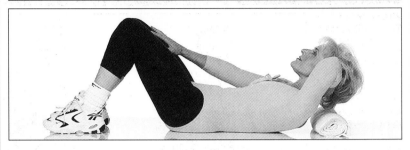

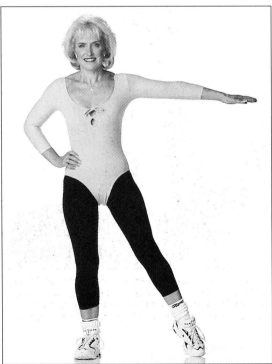

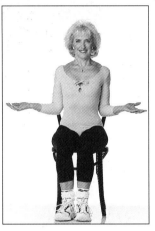

SEQUENCE 3

▲ **16a Box Step with Arms**
As you step forward on the right foot, take the right arm forward at chest height, then follow with the left foot and arm. As you step back, bring each arm back to the hips. You should step wider and deeper now as you need to work harder. Complete 4 complete box steps before moving on to 16b.

◀ **16b Half Jacks with Single Arm** Now take the right toe to touch out at the side, pushing the arm out in the same direction. Bring the feet back together and push out to the other side. Bend the supporting leg more and move more strongly. Repeat 8 times to alternate sides before going back to 16a.

Repeat this sequence 5 times to complete your aerobics session.

▲ **17 Easy Curl** Lie on your back, with knees bent, feet flat on the floor, and your head resting on a rolled-up towel. Adopt the pelvic tilt position by pulling in your tummy and flattening it against the spine. With your left hand behind your head and the other hand resting on the right leg, gently lift your head and shoulders off the floor, keeping your chin off your chest, then lower again. Perform 4 times, breathing out as you lift and breathing in as you lower. Rest and repeat.

◀ **18 Posture Squeezes** Sit upright on a chair, with your feet flat on the floor, and place your elbows close to your waist, with your forearms out in front and your palms facing up, as if you were holding a tray. Now gently take your forearms out to the sides as shown to feel your shoulder blades squeeze closer together at the back. Hold momentarily, then release. Keep it slow and smooth. Do 4, then rest and repeat.

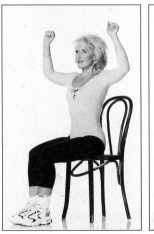
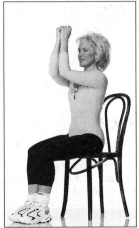

19 Chest Toner Sitting towards the edge of a chair, with your feet flat on the floor, bring your arms out to the sides so that each arm forms a 90-degree angle at chest height. Now squeeze the elbows towards each other, keeping them in line with the chest. Breathe out as you bring them in, and breathe in as you open them again. Perform slowly and smoothly 6 times, then rest and repeat.

20 Underarm Toner Still sitting on the chair, with feet flat on the floor and the trunk upright, take your elbows as far behind you as you can and lean forward slightly. Keep your elbows back as you extend your arms behind. Do 6 slowly, then rest and repeat.

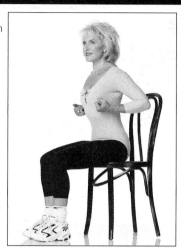
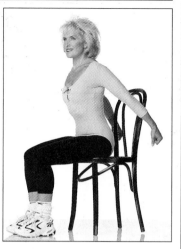

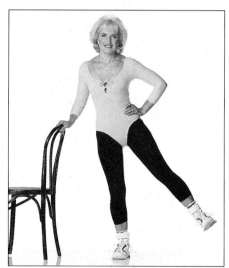

21 Standing Outer Thigh Lift Standing side-on to the chair, place one hand on the chair for support and other hand on your hip. Keep the body upright and, with the leg nearest the chair slightly bent, lift the outside leg off the floor without leaning towards the chair. Lower again, then lift and lower 8 times before turning around to change legs and repeat.

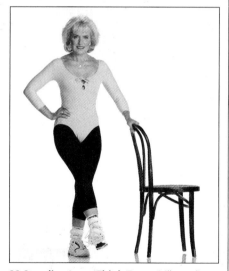

22 Standing Inner Thigh Toner Still standing side-on to the chair, take your weight on to the inside leg. Now, keeping the body upright, draw the outside leg up and across the front of the body, then lower it again. The supporting leg should stay soft. Repeat 8 times, lifting and lowering under control. Turn around to repeat on the other leg.

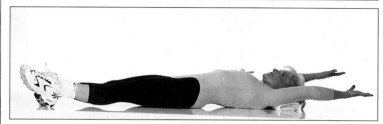

23 Full Body Stretch Lie on your back and take both arms overhead, stretching the legs away from you at the same time. Reach the arms as far away from the legs as is comfortable. Hold for 6 seconds then release.

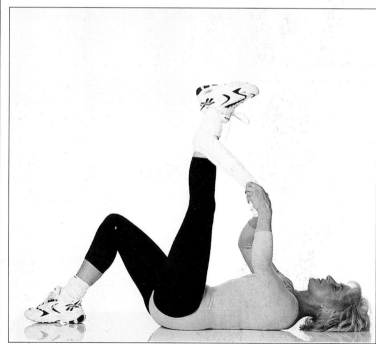

24 Back of Thigh Stretch Lie on your back, with knees bent and feet flat on the floor. Now take hold behind one leg, using a towel to assist, and ease the leg towards the chest. Try to keep the leg as straight as possible, with both hips remaining on the floor, to feel a stretch at the back of the thigh. Hold for 10 seconds, then change legs and repeat.

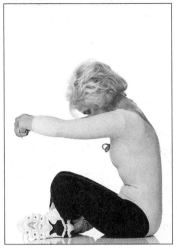

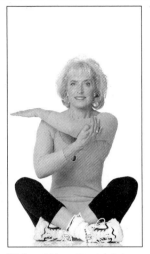

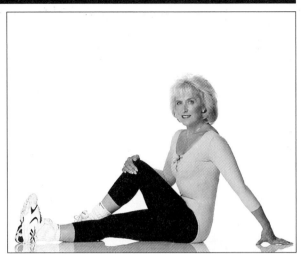

25 Upper Back Stretch Sit cross-legged on the floor and bring your arms forward at chest height. Gently lower your head and press your arms further away from the upper back to feel the stretch across your shoulders. Hold for 8 seconds.

26 Easy Tricep Stretch Bring one arm across in front of the chest. Place the other hand at the back of the upper arm and gently press further across to feel a stretch in the underarm area. Hold for 6 seconds, then change arms and repeat.

27 Outer Thigh Stretch Sit upright, with both legs out in front. Now take your bent right leg across the left knee, using the left hand to press it further across the body and placing the other hand on the floor for support. Hold for 8 seconds, then change legs and repeat.

28 Inner Thigh Stretch Sit with the soles of the feet together and hold your ankles with your hands. Try to place the elbows on the inside of the knees and press down gently to encourage them further toward the floor, and feel the stretch in the inner thigh area. Hold for 10 seconds.

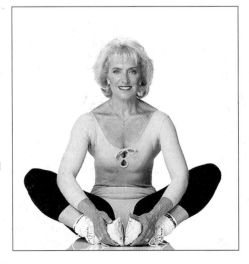

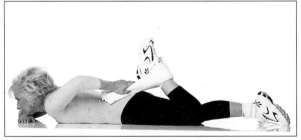

29 Front of Thigh Stretch Lie on your front, with your hands resting under your chin. Now, using your right hand, take hold of the right ankle (you can use a towel to assist if you find this difficult). Bring the heel close to the hip and push the hip down gently into the floor. Hold for 10 seconds, then change legs and repeat.

POSITIVE THOUGHT FOR THE DAY

Congratulations! This is almost the end of Week 1 and you have nearly done it. You are virtually 25 per cent of the way to your new shape and tomorrow morning you will be measuring and weighing yourself. This is a very critical day as you may be feeling a sense of relaxation because you have got this far. It is particularly important that you don't go out and celebrate yet! For some inexplicable reason there seems to be a connection between weighing-in time and bingeing. Ladies often come to my classes and explain that they have been very good all week and yet had a binge just prior to the class! It is a psychological battle that we sometimes have to wage. So please stick at the programme until tomorrow morning.

Don't eat rice or pasta today. Try to stick to the suggested menu and have your main meal at lunchtime. This gives your body more time to burn up the calories. Be as active as possible. I promise you'll be glad tomorrow. Best of luck!

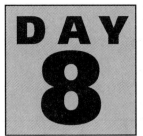

DAY 8

This is a really important day. Before you step on the scales, find your tape measure and record your measurements on the Weight and Inch Loss Record Chart at the back of this book. Measure yourself before you eat or drink anything to get your most accurate reading.

As mentioned earlier, scales can sometimes show disappointing results because of fluid fluctuations within the body. The tape measure is a much more accurate way of assessing your progress. If you have lost pounds too, all the better.

Today treat yourself to your favourite menus of the last week – any breakfast, lunch or dinner – or try my special menu designed to mark your achievement so far.

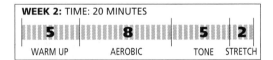

WEEK 2: TIME: 20 MINUTES

5	8	5	2
WARM UP	AEROBIC	TONE	STRETCH

— Menu —

BREAKFAST

25g (1oz) any cereal of your choice with 1 small banana, served with milk from allowance and 1 teaspoon of sugar

OR

115g (4oz) fresh fruit salad and 1 × 150g (5oz) diet yogurt

LUNCH

4 slices of light bread (max 200kcals) spread with reduced-oil salad dressing and made into sandwiches with 75g (3oz) salmon or tuna (in brine), cucumber and tomatoes, plus ½ a fresh grapefruit

OR

5 Ryvitas spread with low-calorie coleslaw and topped with sliced tomatoes, lettuce and cucumber, plus 1 × 150g (5oz) diet yogurt

DINNER

CHICKEN CHINESE STYLE (see recipe, page 175)
PLUS
1 meringue basket filled with fresh or frozen raspberries topped with low-fat raspberry fromage frais

OR

SWEETCORN AND POTATO FRITTERS
(see recipe, page 184)
served with RATATOUILLE (see recipe, page 181)
and peas
PLUS
HOT CHERRIES (see recipe, page 178)

Today you are allowed an extra glass of wine or champagne to celebrate the achievement of completing your first week.

WARM UP – MOBILITY AND PULSE-RAISING

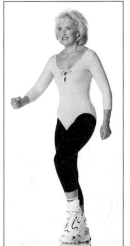

The mobility and pulse-raising sections are now combined so that you can really get moving as you warm up.

1 March on the Spot
Stand tall, with your head up and shoulders back, and march on the spot, really picking the knees up and swinging the arms. Make sure the heels go down to the floor with each step. March for 32 counts, counting 1 for every alternate step.

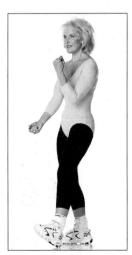
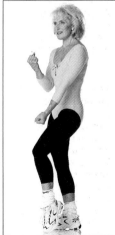

2 Heel/Toe with Bicep Curls Take the right heel out diagonally in front on the floor and then change to the toe. At the same time bend alternate elbows, keeping them close to the waist and under control. Rhythmically keep changing from heel to toe for 4 counts, counting 1 every time the heel strikes the floor. Change legs and repeat, then repeat again on each leg.

3 Half Jacks with Single Arm Starting with feet together, take one leg and one arm out to the side, touching just the toe to the floor. Bring them back to the middle and do the same on the other side. Stand tall throughout and make sure the supporting knee remains slightly bent. Keep changing sides for 16 counts.

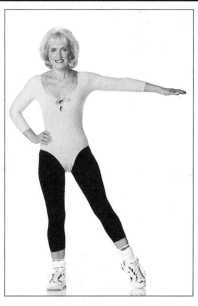

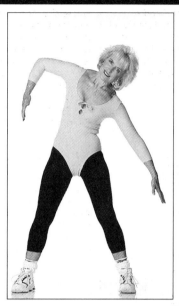

4 Side Bends Stand with feet apart and knees slightly bent. Now lean over to the right side, reaching out with the right arm and lifting the left elbow up. Come up to the centre and then lean to the other side. Keep the hips still throughout and try not to lean forward or back. Repeat 12 times altogether, changing sides each time.

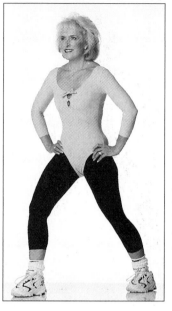

All the stretches are now performed standing. If you find it difficult to balance, then use a wall to help support you.

7 Calf Stretch Stand with one foot in front of the other, with the front leg bent and the back leg straight. Keep your tummy in and your head up and lean forward slightly to feel the stretch in the lower leg at the back. Hold for 6 seconds, then change legs and repeat.

5 Touch Backs Start with feet together, then take one foot behind you, touching the floor with just the toe. At the same time reach both arms forward to chest height. You can lean forward slightly but make sure your tummy is in tight to support your back. Keep changing legs and repeat 12 times altogether.

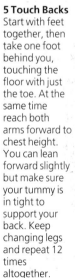

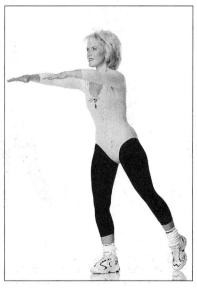

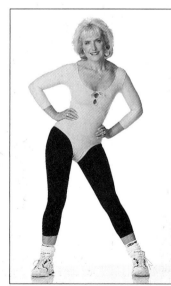

6 Hip Rolls With feet wide apart and knees bent, roll the hips around in a full circle, from the side, round to the front, and then to the back. Keep it very smooth and under control. Repeat 4 times slowly in one direction, then change direction and repeat.

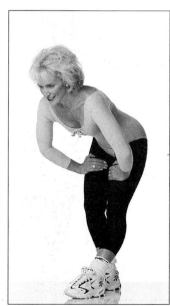

8 Back of Thigh Stretch Stand with your back leg bent and your front leg straight, and place your hands in the middle of your thighs. Now, keeping your head up and your back flat, lean forward until you feel a stretch in the back of the straight leg. Hold for 6 seconds, then change legs and repeat.

9 Inner Thigh Stretch Take the legs very wide and place one foot out diagonally, with the knee bent in line with the toes. The other leg is straight, with the foot pointing forward. To feel the stretch on the inside of the thigh, take the straight leg further away from you. Hold for 6 seconds, then change legs and repeat.

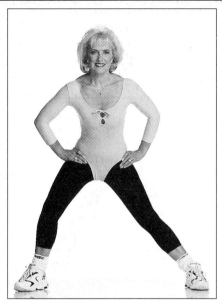

11 Front of Thigh Stretch Take hold around one ankle so that the knee points towards the floor and the knees are fairly close together. Try to keep the knee of the supporting leg slightly bent and push the hip forward on the held leg to feel the stretch down the front of the thigh. Hold for 6 seconds, then change legs and repeat.

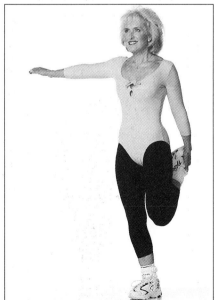

10 Chest Stretch Stand with feet slightly apart and your head up. Now place your hands in the small of your back and squeeze your elbows back behind you to feel a stretch across the chest. Hold for 6 seconds, then release.

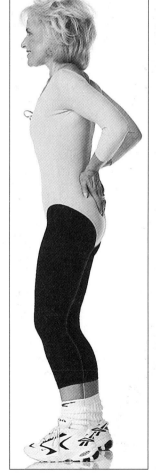

This session is now longer to increase your fat-burning potential. Try to learn the sequences so that you do not need to refer to the text, and work out to a favourite piece of music that you can comfortably march to. The arms are included in every move. However, if you want to keep moving but work at a lower intensity, simply take out the arm movements.

SEQUENCE 1

12a Step Touch Swing Step from side to side, swinging your arms to just above chest height. Make the steps wide and bend your knees well as you step out. Keep your head up and your back lifted. Repeat 8 times before moving on to 12b.

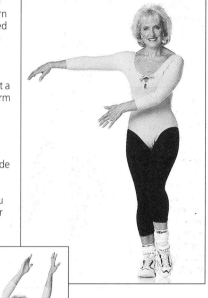

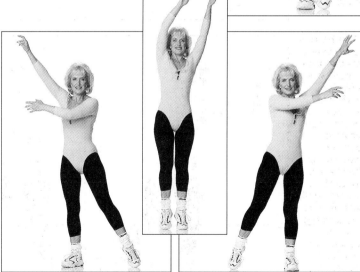

12b Travel Overs Now take 2 steps to the right, taking your arms over in a circular motion in front of you. Then take 2 steps to the left, letting your arms swing naturally over the top. Repeat twice through to each side then go back to 12a.

Repeat this sequence 4 times.

SEQUENCE 2

13a Hopscotch with Elbow Presses Step out to the side with the right leg and bend the left knee up behind you. At the same time your arms are up at chest height and the elbows press behind you as you lift the leg. Keep your body upright, tummy pulled in tightly and keep the knee of the supporting leg slightly bent. Do 8 hopscotches before changing to 13b.

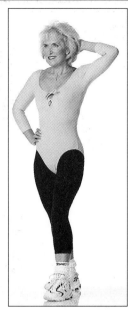 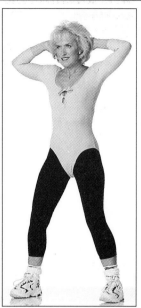 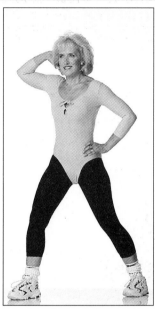 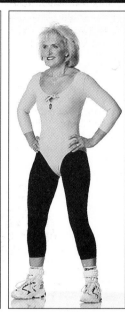

13b Walks with Rolling Arms Walk forward for 3 counts, stop on the 4th count and clap your hands. Now do the same thing but moving backwards. Try to roll your arms up at chest height as you walk. Repeat forward and back twice before going back to 13a.

Repeat this sequence 4 times.

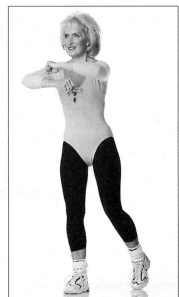 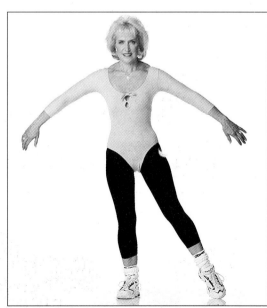

SEQUENCE 3

▲ **14a Box Step with Funky Arms** Take one step forward and out with the right foot, placing your right hand at the side of your head at the same time. Now take the other foot forward, placing your left hand on your head. As you step back on the right, bring that hand back to the hip, then do the same on the left. Keep stepping forward and back rhythmically 4 times before changing to 14b.

◄ **14b Half Jacks with Arms** Start with your feet together, then tap the right toe out to the side, taking both arms out to the sides at the same time. Bring the feet together again and change to the other side. Keep changing from side to side for 8 repetitions, then go back to 14a.

Repeat this sequence 4 times, then repeat each sequence once more to complete this aerobics session.

Each muscle is made to work harder this week, so the positions you have adopted before have changed, and, in some cases, you will do more repetitions. If any exercise becomes too uncomfortable, always go back to the easy position and take a rest when you need to.

▼ **15 Abdominal Curl** Lie on your back and place a towel under your head for comfort if you wish. Bend both knees, with your feet flat on the floor and your tummy pulled well in against the spine. Place one hand behind your head and the other hand across your chest. Now gently lift your head and shoulders off the floor, then lower again. Repeat 6 times slowly, breathing out as you lift and breathing in as you lower again. Rest and repeat.

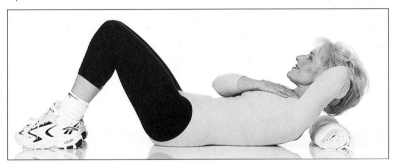

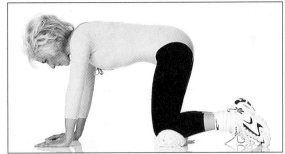

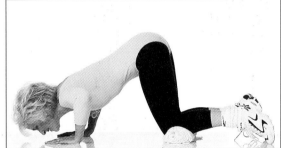

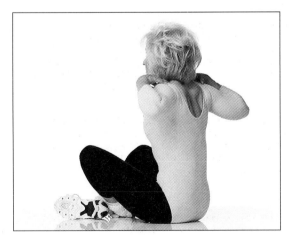

17 Posture Improver Sit up, with your legs comfortably crossed. Keeping your head up and your back straight, place your hands on your shoulders. Now squeeze your shoulders back slowly and under control, then release. Repeat 4 times, then rest and do 4 more.

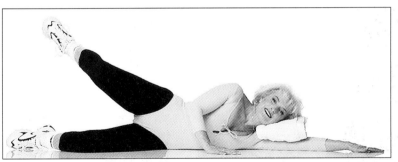

16 Press Ups Come up onto your hands and knees, with your hands under your shoulders and your knees under your hips. If you wish, you can place a towel under your knees to release any pressure. Now, keeping your tummy pulled in tight to protect the spine, slowly take your forehead down towards the floor in front of your hands, then press back up again without locking the elbows at the top. Repeat 4 times slowly, then rest and repeat.

18 Outer Thigh Toner Lie on your side, with your arm extended and your head resting comfortably on a towel. Bend both legs so that each forms a 45-degree angle. Now lift the top leg to just above hip height, keeping the hips stacked on top of each other, then lower under control. Repeat 8 times, then change to the other leg.

19 Bottom Toner Lie on your front, with your head resting on your hands and the towel positioned under your hips. Gently lift one leg, keeping it straight and keeping your hips facing the floor. Keep alternating legs for 8 repetitions, then rest and repeat.

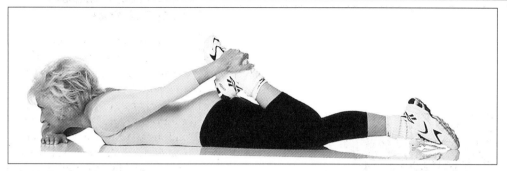

20 Front of Thigh Stretch Lie on your front, bend your right knee up and take hold of the ankle. Ease the heel close to the hip and push that hip firmly into the floor. Hold for 10 seconds, then change legs and repeat.

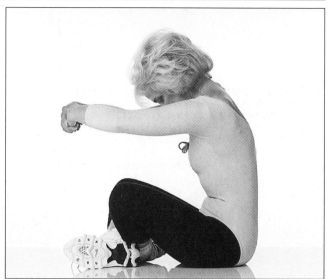

▶ **21 Upper Back Stretch** Sit cross-legged, bring both arms round in front of you at chest height and clasp your hands. Drop your head forward, and round your spine to feel a stretch across the back of the shoulders. Hold for 8 seconds, then release.

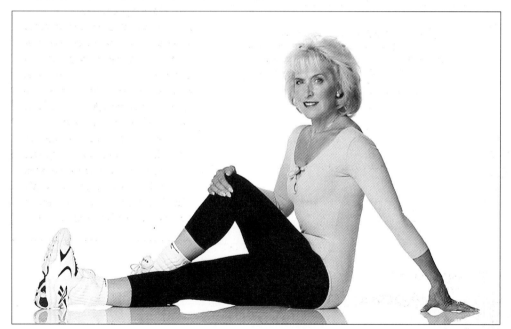

22 Outer Thigh Stretch Sit with both legs out in front, then cross your right leg over the left and place your right foot in line with the left knee. Now place your left hand on the outside of the right knee and the other hand on the floor for support. Gently squeeze the right knee further across the chest to feel a stretch in the outer thigh. Hold for 8 seconds, then release. Change legs and repeat.

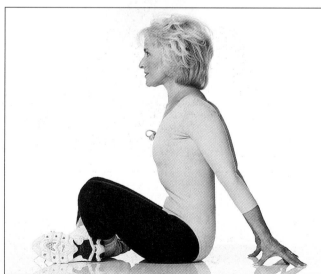

23 Chest Stretch Sit cross-legged and place your hands behind you on the floor. Now, sitting upright, squeeze the shoulders back to feel a stretch across the chest. Hold for 8 seconds, then release.

▶ 24a Bottom Stretch Lie on your back, with both knees bent and feet flat on the floor. Draw one knee into the chest, holding underneath the knee, and squeeze the raised leg towards the chest to feel a stretch in your bottom. Hold for 10 seconds, then move on to 24b.

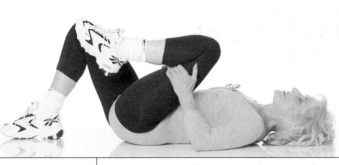

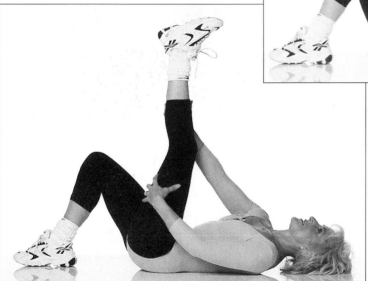

◀ 24b Back of Thigh Stretch Now extend the leg further to feel the stretch move to the back of the thigh. Keep your hips on the floor and move one hand further up the leg for support. Hold for 10 seconds, then try to extend the knee a little further in order to develop the stretch more. Hold for a further 10 seconds, then release.

Repeat 24a and 24b on the other leg.

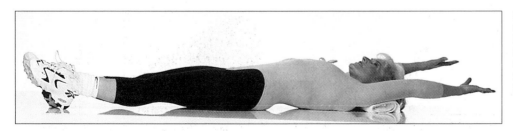

25 Full Body Stretch Lie on your back and take both arms over your head as you extend both legs away from you. Hold for 8 seconds, then slowly release.

POSITIVE THOUGHT FOR THE DAY

I hope you feel that you are really making progress. The exercises are becoming increasingly effective as your body becomes more acclimatised to the actions. Your muscles are now being challenged and this will create a much more beautiful body shape. Take the time to look at yourself in the mirror and recognise the improvements.

Today I would like you to take a small piece of card which you will keep for your eyes only. On it I would like you to write:

I am much slimmer and a better shape than I have been for some time (or for months, years, etc.) and I am going to get even slimmer and achieve an even better figure – a figure I never thought I could have. This time I know I can do it!

Please take the trouble to write this or a similar message and look at it often. Picture yourself succeeding. If you can honestly visualise yourself as you want to be, you cannot fail to achieve it!

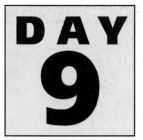

DAY 9

Did you enjoy yesterday? I hope you are feeling more energetic as you become fitter and slimmer each day.

How are you getting on with the exercises? Remember, only do what you can – please don't over-exert yourself. You are not training for the next Olympics, just getting a little fitter and making your heart work more efficiently and become stronger.

Try on your measuring skirt/trousers again today. It will definitely be feeling looser. Doesn't it feel good!

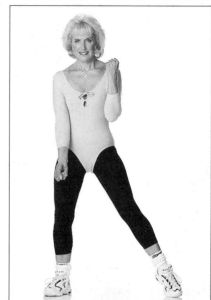

1 Step Touch with Bicep Curls
Stand tall and step out to alternate sides, bending your knees as the feet come together. At the same time bend alternate elbows, keeping them close to the waist. Perform 16 times altogether.

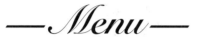

—Menu—

BREAKFAST

2 turkey rashers, grilled or dry-fried, served with 115g (4oz) tinned tomatoes and 115g (4oz) mushrooms, grilled or dry-fried

OR

25g (1oz) Kellogg's All-Bran mixed with 15g (½oz) muesli and served with milk from allowance and 1 teaspoon of sugar

LUNCH

5 brown Ryvitas topped with SALAD SURPRISE (see recipe, page 182), plus 1 piece of fresh fruit or 1 × 150g (5oz) diet yogurt

OR

Jacket potato (any size) topped with 115g (4oz) baked beans and 50g (2oz) sweetcorn, plus 1 × 150g (5oz) diet yogurt

DINNER

115g (4oz) chicken (no skin) served with unlimited vegetables and a little gravy
PLUS
MELON SURPRISE
(see recipe, page 179)

OR

VEGETARIAN CHILLI CON CARNE
(see recipe, page 185)
PLUS
CHEESE PEARS (see recipe, page 175)

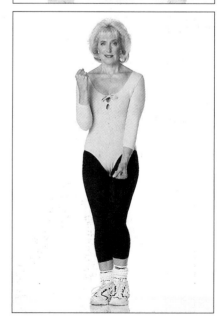

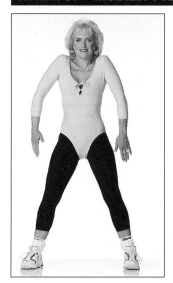

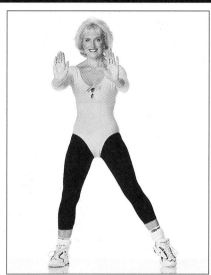

4 Waist Twists
Stand upright, with feet apart, tummy pulled in and knees slightly bent. Now place your hands on your shoulders and twist round as far as you can go, keeping the hips facing forward. Return to face front and do the same to the other side. Keep it smooth and controlled. Do 12, changing sides each time.

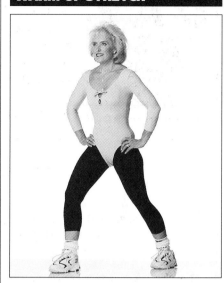

2 Double Shoulder Lifts Standing with feet apart, shoulders back and head up, smoothly raise both shoulders up toward the ears, then press them down again. Perform 8 times under control.

3 Double Steps with Arm Presses Take 2 steps to the right and, at the same time, press both arms out in front at chest height. Now take 2 steps back to the left. Keep your body upright, with your shoulders back and your head up. Repeat the sequence 4 times altogether.

7 Calf Stretch Stand with one foot in front of the other, with the front leg bent and the back leg straight. Keep your tummy in and your head up and lean forward slightly to feel the stretch in the lower leg at the back. Hold for 6 seconds, then change legs and repeat.

5 Touch Backs with Arms
Start with feet together, then take one foot behind you, touching the floor with just the toe. At the same time reach both arms forward to chest height. You can lean forward slightly but make sure your tummy is in tight to support your back. Keep changing legs, and repeat 12 times altogether.

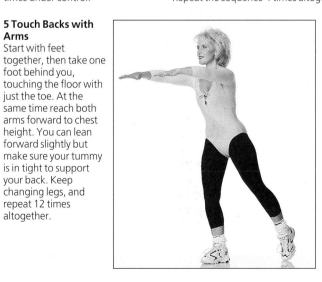

6 Knee Bends with Wide Arms Stand with legs wide apart and feet turned out slightly. Now bend your knees in line with the toes, taking your hips back as if you were trying to sit in a chair. At the same time, bring both arms out to the sides to shoulder height. Come up without locking the knees fully, bringing the arms back down to your sides. Repeat 8 times slowly.

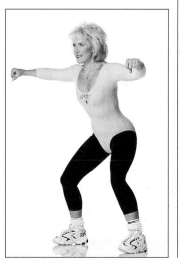

8 Back of Thigh Stretch Stand with your back leg bent and your front leg straight, and place your hands in the middle of your thighs. Now, keeping your head up and your back flat, lean forward until you feel a stretch in the back of the straight leg. Hold for 6 seconds, then change legs and repeat.

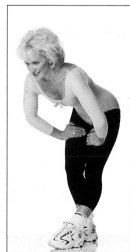

9 Waist Stretch Stand with feet apart, place your right hand on your shoulder and place your left hand at the top of your left thigh for support. Now gently lean to the left until you feel the right elbow is pointing up to the ceiling to feel a stretch down the waist. Hold for 6 seconds, then change sides and repeat.

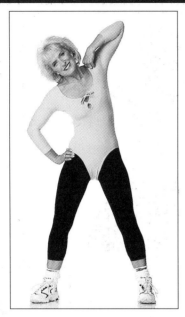

10 Inner Thigh Stretch Take the legs very wide and place one foot out diagonally, with the knee bent in line with the toes. The other leg is straight, with the foot pointing forward. To feel the stretch on the inside of the thigh, take the straight leg further away from you. Hold for 6 seconds, then change legs and repeat.

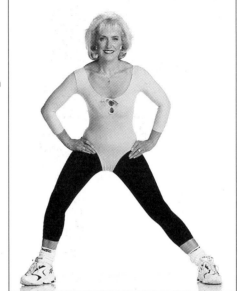

11 Chest Stretch Stand with feet slightly apart and your head up. Now place your hands in the small of your back and squeeze your elbows back behind you to feel a stretch across the chest. Hold for 6 seconds, then release.

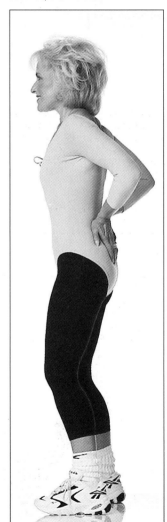

12 Tricep Stretch Stand with feet apart, tummy pulled in tight and knees slightly bent. Now take your right hand behind the right shoulder and use the left hand on the fleshy part of the right underarm to push it further back. Keep your head up throughout and hold for 6 seconds. Change arms and repeat.

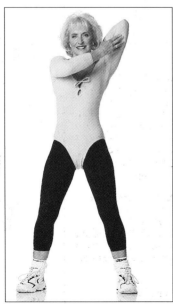

13 Front of Thigh Stretch Take hold around one ankle so that the knee points towards the floor and the knees are fairly close together. Try to keep the knee of the supporting leg slightly bent and push the hip forward on the held leg to feel the stretch down the front of the thigh. Hold for 6 seconds, then change legs and repeat.

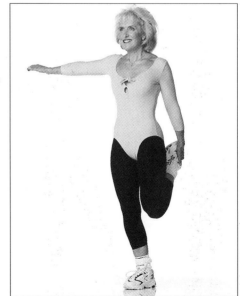

SEQUENCE 1

▶ **14a Step Touch Swing** Step from side to side, swinging your arms to just above chest height. Make the steps wide and bend your knees well as you step out. Keep your head up and your back lifted. Repeat 8 times before moving on to 14b.

▼ **14b Travel Overs** Now take 2 steps to the right, taking your arms over in a circular motion in front of you. Then take 2 steps to the left, letting your arms swing naturally over the top. Repeat twice through to each side then go back to 14a.

Repeat this sequence 4 times.

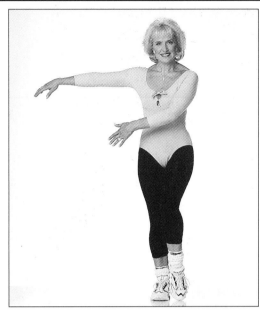

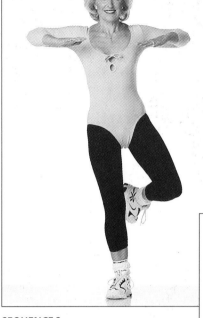

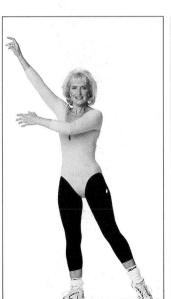

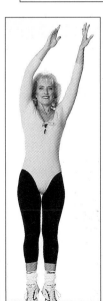

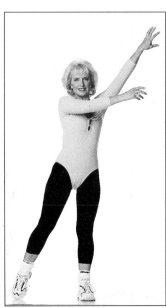

SEQUENCE 2

▲ **15a Hopscotch with Elbow Presses** Step out to the side with the right leg and bend the left knee up behind you. At the same time your arms are up at chest height and the elbows press behind you as you lift the leg. Keep your body upright, tummy pulled in tightly and keep the knee of the supporting leg slightly bent. Do 8 hopscotches before changing to 15b.

▶ **15b Walks with Rolling Arms** Walk forward for 3 counts, stop on the 4th count and clap your hands. Now do the same thing but moving backwards. Try to roll your arms up at chest height as you walk. Repeat forward and back twice before going back to 15a.

Repeat this sequence 4 times.

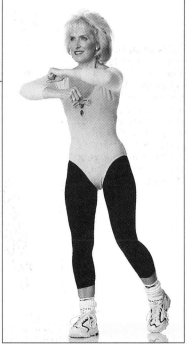

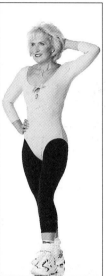

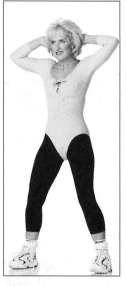

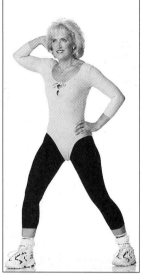

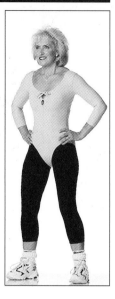

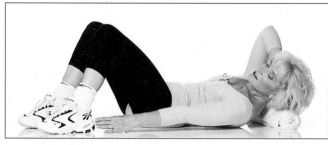

17 Waist Reach Lie on your back, with your knees bent and feet flat on the floor. Place a rolled towel under your head and place your right hand behind your head. Use your left hand to reach round towards your left ankle, with your head slightly raised. Come back to the centre and swap hands to reach down the other side. Keep your tummy pulled in tight against your spine and keep the movement slow and controlled. Repeat 4 times to each side, then rest and repeat.

SEQUENCE 3

▲ **16a Box Step with Funky Arms** Take one step forward and out with the right foot, placing your right hand at the side of your head at the same time. Now take the other foot forward, placing your left hand on your head. As you step back on the right, bring that hand back to the hip, then do the same on the left. Keep stepping forward and back rhythmically 4 times before changing to 16b.

◄ **16b Half Jacks with Arms** Start with your feet together, then tap the right toe out to the side, taking both arms out to the sides at the same time. Bring the feet together again and change to the other side. Keep changing from side to side for 8 repetitions, then go back to 16a.

Repeat this sequence 4 times, then repeat each sequence once more to complete this aerobics session.

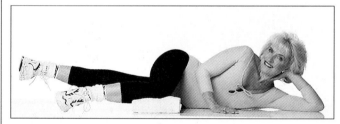

18 Inner Thigh Toner Lie on your side, with your head in your hand, or you can lie right down on your arm if it is more comfortable. Bring the top leg over the underneath leg and rest the knee on the towel. Now lift the underneath leg just off the floor, keeping the foot pulled towards you. Lift and lower under control 8 times, then change legs and repeat.

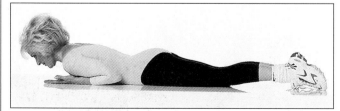

19 Back Raises Lie on your front, with your elbows close to your waist and the palms up. Keep looking at the floor as you slowly lift the upper body about 7.5cm (3in) from the floor, and lower again. Keep both feet firmly on the floor. Repeat 4 times, breathing out as you lift and breathing in as you lower. Rest and repeat.

20 Press Ups
Come up onto your hands and knees, with your hands under your shoulders and your knees under your hips. If you wish, you can place a towel under your knees to release any pressure. Now, keeping your tummy pulled in tight to protect the spine, slowly take your forehead down towards the floor in front of your hands, then press back up again without locking the elbows at the top. Repeat 4 times slowly, then rest and repeat.

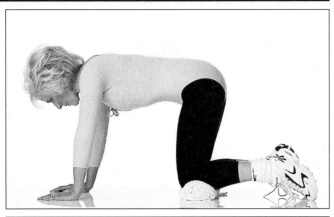

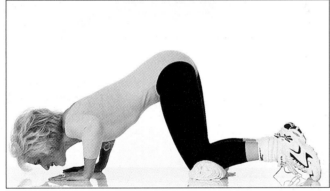

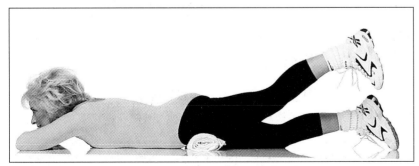

21 Bottom Toner Lie on your front, with your head resting on your hands and the towel positioned under your hips. Gently lift one leg, keeping it straight and keeping your hips facing the floor. Keep alternating legs for 8 repetitions, then rest and repeat.

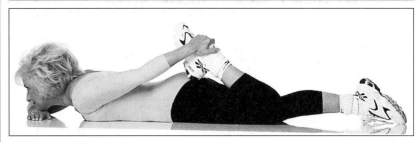

22 Front of Thigh Stretch Lie on your front, bend your right knee up and take hold of the ankle. Ease the heel close to the hip and push that hip firmly into the floor. Hold for 10 seconds, then change legs and repeat.

23 Spine Stretch Come up into a box shape on hands and knees. Now pull your tummy in tightly, arching your back and tucking your hips under. Hold for 8 seconds, then release.

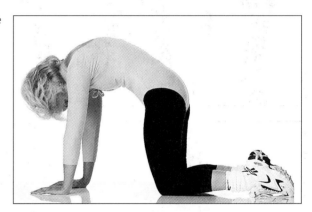

24 Chest Stretch Sit upright, with legs comfortably crossed. Now place your hands on the floor behind you and gently lift up from the base of the spine, squeezing the shoulder blades together at the back. Hold for 6 seconds, then release.

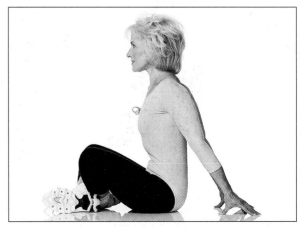

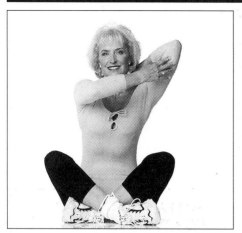

25 Underarm Stretch Sitting with legs crossed, head up and shoulders back, place your right hand behind your right shoulder and take the left hand across in front to push the arm further back. Hold for 6 seconds, then change sides and repeat.

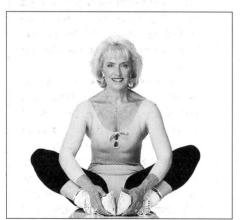

26 Inner Thigh Stretch Sit with soles of the feet together and your hands around your ankles. Now sit up tall and, with a straight back, lean forward slightly to place the elbows on to the inside of the knees. Press down gently to feel a stretch on the inside of the thighs. Hold for 10 seconds, then try to press further to develop the stretch more. Hold for 5 more seconds, then release.

27a Bottom Stretch Lie on your back, with both knees bent and feet flat on the floor. Draw one knee into the chest, holding underneath the knee, and squeeze the raised leg towards the chest to feel a stretch in your bottom. Hold for 10 seconds, then move on to 27b.

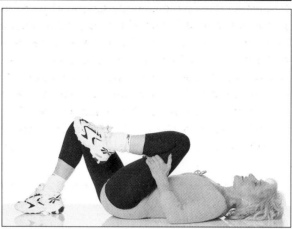

27b Back of Thigh Stretch Now extend the leg further to feel the stretch move to the back of the thigh. Keep your hips on the floor and move one hand further up the leg for support. Hold for 10 seconds, then try to extend the knee a little further in order to develop the stretch more. Hold for a further 10 seconds, then release.

Repeat 27a and 27b on the other leg.

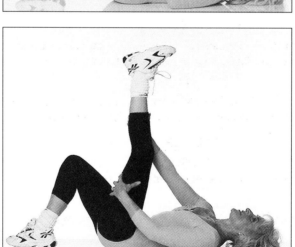

28 Full Body Stretch Lie on your back and take both arms over your head as you extend both legs away from you. Hold for 8 seconds, then slowly release.

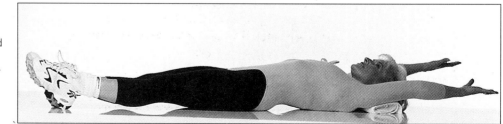

POSITIVE THOUGHT FOR THE DAY

You should now be looking significantly slimmer and will no doubt be attracting some comments – hopefully, complimentary ones. There will, however, always be those who tend to see the negative side and may well suggest you don't lose weight too quickly or 'you'll look old' or 'you'll only put it back on twice as fast if you lose it quickly'. These so-called friends are usually overweight, failed dieters who can't bear to see you succeeding. What she (or he) doesn't realise is that you won't have actually lost very much weight (perhaps 2lb or 3lb), but you will look much slimmer because you are holding yourself so much better and have lost inches. Always try to respond positively to negative comments, perhaps by saying 'I've never felt so good for years' – only if it's true, of course.

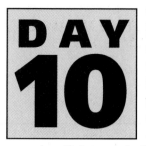

DAY 10

Well, it's now 10 days into your 28-day programme and you should be seeing some real results. Selecting low-fat foods in the supermarket or food store, and cooking and serving food without fat has now become a habit, and I expect you are feeling that you don't miss the fat at all, particularly as you see the inches dropping away from you. Nothing succeeds like success, so don't be self-conscious about looking at yourself in the mirror and seeing your progress for yourself. Remember to maintain a good posture at all times. We have a built-in Playtex girdle – the transverse muscle – which lies underneath our other abdominal muscles. This muscle can be contracted at all times and will significantly help your stomach to look flatter and help you adopt a better posture.

Take another rest day from the exercises today, but stay active. Enjoy your meals today and watch those pounds and inches diminish still further.

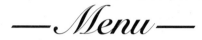

BREAKFAST

Mix 1 tablespoon of jam or honey into 115g (4oz) low-fat cottage cheese or
225g (8oz) low-fat fromage frais or Total 0% Greek yogurt

OR

1 slice of wholemeal toast topped with 400g (14oz) tinned tomatoes boiled well and reduced
to a creamy consistency to prevent the toast becoming soggy

LUNCH

INCH LOSS SALAD
(see recipe, page 178), served with chicken or prawns

OR

4 pieces of any fresh fruit plus 1 × 150g (5oz) diet yogurt

DINNER

FISH CAKES (see recipe, page 176)
PLUS
1 slice of KIM'S CAKE
(see recipe, page 178) and 1 × 150g (5oz) diet yogurt

OR

1 × 350g pack of Marks & Spencer Spinach Ricotta Cannelloni
PLUS
1 Marks & Spencer Lite Mousse, any flavour

POSITIVE THOUGHT FOR THE DAY

Confidence is a wonderful thing — it creates the courage we need to open up all kinds of doors. Would you like to feel totally happy with yourself and able to cope with any situation without feeling inadequate? Would you like to feel every bit as good as the next person?

Think of someone whom you admire at the moment. What is it about them that makes them stand out from the rest? At some stage in their lives they decided they were going to be a winner not a loser. Instead of saying 'I can't do that' or 'I'm no good at that' they switched to 'I could have a go at that' and then 'well, if they can do that, why shouldn't I? Today I want you to turn that corner and change from a feeling of 'I'm never going to do it' to 'I will do it'.

Did you feel more positive about your future when you woke up this morning? Do you feel totally confident about achieving the figure you want?

Do you remember making all the usual excuses about being overweight? 'I was a big baby, so I'm obviously meant to be this size – all my family are big' or 'I've tried diet after diet, they just don't seem to work for me' or 'I only have to look at a cream cake and I gain 2lb'. These are all negative personal conditioning statements. If we say them often enough we will actually believe them and make them happen. No wonder we've failed previously! Instead, we are now saying 'I know this diet and exercise plan is working for me. This time I am going to reach my weight and inch loss goal because I never feel hungry and I am eating the foods I enjoy, I don't even feel as though I'm dieting. This will be the last time I have to diet because I have a completely different attitude towards my body and the food that I eat'.

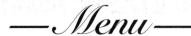

—Menu—

BREAKFAST

20g (³/₄oz) bran flakes mixed with 25g (1oz) sultanas and served with milk from allowance, no sugar

OR

115g (4oz) tinned peaches in natural juice and 1 × 150g (5oz) diet yogurt

LUNCH

3 brown Ryvitas or 50g (2oz) wholemeal bread spread with 75g (3oz) pilchards or sardines in tomato sauce topped with sliced tomatoes and salad, plus 1 banana

OR

225g (8oz) low-fat cottage cheese with a chopped pear, chopped apple and 2 sticks celery, chopped, served on a bed of lettuce, tomatoes and cucumber

DINNER

75g (3oz) roast leg of pork (with all fat removed) served with 50g (2oz) apple sauce, 115g (4oz) DRY-ROAST POTATOES (see recipe, page 176) and unlimited vegetables
PLUS
115g (4oz) fresh fruit salad topped with 1 × 150g (5oz) diet yogurt

OR

Marks & Spencer Healthy Choice Low Fat Cauliflower Cheese, plus 115g (4oz) potatoes and unlimited vegetables
PLUS
115g (4oz) stewed fruit topped with 1 × 150g (5oz) appropriate flavoured diet yogurt

WARM UP – MOBILITY AND PULSE-RAISING

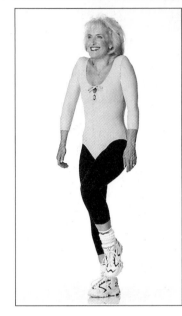

1 March on the Spot with Shoulder Lifts
Stand up straight, with your head up and your shoulders back, and march on the spot. As you march, lift both shoulders up towards your ears and then down again, keeping the action slow and controlled. Lift the shoulders for 2 marches and then lower them for 2 to keep a rhythmical pace. Lift and lower the shoulders 8 times altogether.

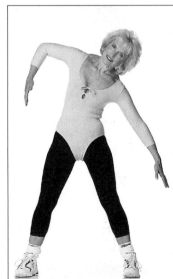

2 Side Bends
Stand with feet apart and knees slightly bent. Now lean over to the right side, reaching out with the right arm and lifting the left elbow up. Come up to the centre and then lean to the other side. Keep the hips still throughout and try not to lean forward or back. Repeat 12 times altogether, changing sides each time.

3 Neck Mobiliser
Stand with feet apart, tummy in and shoulders back. Now slowly turn your head to the right, keeping the shoulders facing front. Return to the centre and repeat to the other side. Repeat only 3 times to each side.

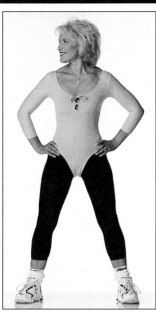

4 Double Steps with Arm Presses
Take 2 steps to the right and, at the same time, press both arms out in front at chest height. Now take 2 steps back to the left. Keep your body upright, with your shoulders back and your head up. Repeat the sequence 4 times altogether.

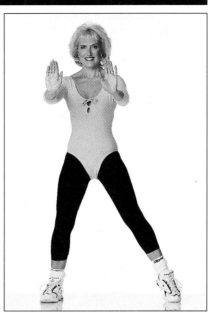

7 Calf Stretch
Stand with one foot in front of the other, with the front leg bent and the back leg straight. Keep your tummy in and your head up and lean forward slightly to feel the stretch in the lower leg at the back. Hold for 6 seconds, then change legs and repeat.

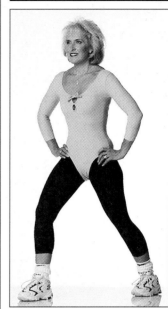

5 Knee Lifts Take a step out to the side with the right leg then lift the left knee up to waist height, keeping your back straight and your head up. Try to touch the raised knee with the opposite hand. Perform 24, alternating legs.

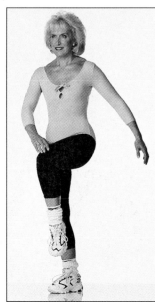

6 Heel/Toe with Bicep Curls Take the right heel out diagonally in front on the floor and then change to the toe. At the same time bend alternate elbows, keeping them close to the waist and under control. Rhythmically keep changing from heel to toe for 4 counts, counting 1 every time the heel strikes the floor. Change legs and repeat, then repeat again on each leg.

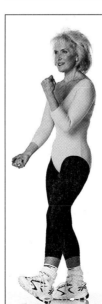
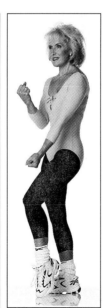

8 Back of Thigh Stretch Stand with your back leg bent and your front leg straight, and place your hands in the middle of your thighs. Now, keeping your head up and your back flat, lean forward until you feel a stretch in the back of the straight leg. Hold for 6 seconds, then change legs and repeat.

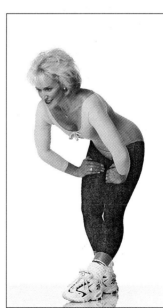

9 Front of Thigh Stretch Take hold around one ankle so that the knee points towards the floor and the knees are fairly close together. Try to keep the knee of the supporting leg slightly bent and push the hip forward on the held leg to feel the stretch down the front of the thigh. Hold for 6 seconds, then change legs and repeat.

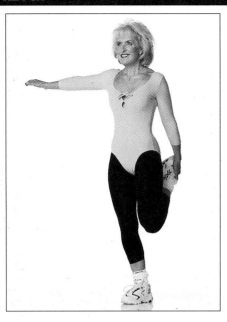

10 Upper Back Stretch Standing with feet comfortably apart, bring your arms round in front of your chest and clasp your hands together. Drop your head forward and gently press the arms away from the hands to feel a stretch across the shoulder blades at the back. Hold for 6 seconds, then release.

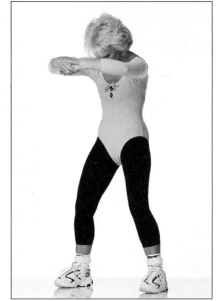

11 Chest Stretch Stand with feet slightly apart and your head up. Now place your hands in the small of your back and squeeze your elbows back behind you to feel a stretch across the chest. Hold for 6 seconds, then release.

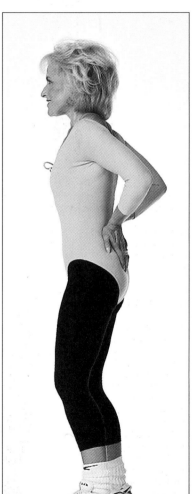

12 Inner Thigh Stretch Take the legs very wide and place one foot out diagonally, with the knee bent in line with the toes. The other leg is straight, with the foot pointing forward. To feel the stretch on the inside of the thigh, take the straight leg further away from you. Hold for 6 seconds, then change legs and repeat.

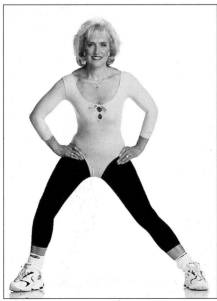

13 Tricep Stretch Stand with feet apart, tummy pulled in tight and knees slightly bent. Now take your right hand behind the right shoulder and use the left hand on the fleshy part of the right underarm to push it further back. Keep your head up throughout and hold for 6 seconds. Change arms and repeat.

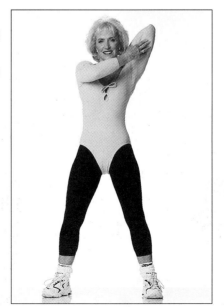

SEQUENCE 1

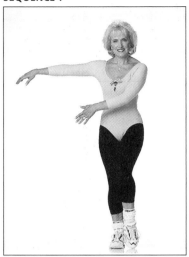
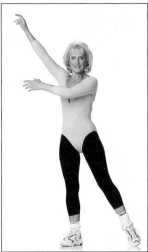
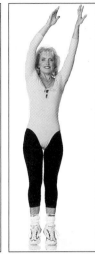
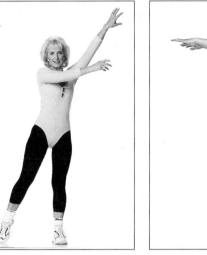
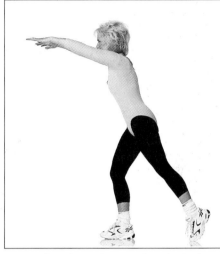

14a Step Touch Swing Step from side to side, swinging your arms to just above chest height. Make the steps wide and bend your knees well as you step out. Keep your head up and your back lifted. Repeat 8 times before moving on to 14b.

14b Travel Overs Now take 2 steps to the right, taking your arms over in a circular motion in front of you. Then take 2 steps to the left, letting your arms swing naturally over the top. Repeat twice through to each side then move on to 14c.

14c Touch Backs On the return from the final travel over take the right toe to touch the floor behind you and push the arms forward at the same time. Lean forward slightly to protect your back, and keep your tummy pulled in tight. Repeat 8 times before going back to the step touch swing to repeat Sequence 1 again.

SEQUENCE 2

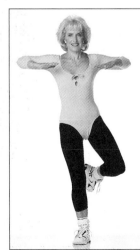

15a Hopscotch with Elbow Presses Step out to the side with the right leg and bend the left knee up behind you. At the same time your arms are up at chest height and the elbows press behind you as you lift the leg. Keep your body upright, tummy pulled in tightly and keep the knee of the supporting leg slightly bent. Do 8 hopscotches before changing to 15b.

15b Walks with Rolling Arms Walk forward for 3 counts, stop on the 4th count and clap your hands. Now do the same thing but moving backwards. Try to roll your arms up at chest height as you walk. Repeat forward and back twice before moving on to 15c.

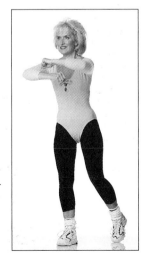

15c Skip Turns On the return from the last walk back, take a turn on the spot all the way round to your right, using a small bouncing skip. Make sure the heels land on the floor on each skip. (If you don't want to skip, you can march instead.) Use 4 counts to turn to the right then another 4 to turn to the left. Now go back to the hopscotch to repeat Sequence 2 again.

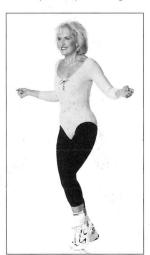

A new move has been added to each sequence to add interest and to motivate you to stick at it!

SEQUENCE 3

16a Box Step with Funky Arms Take one step forward and out with the right foot, placing your right hand at the side of your head at the same time. Now take the other foot forward, placing your left hand on your head. As you step back on the right, bring that hand back to the hip, then do the same on the left. Keep stepping forward and back rhythmically 4 times before changing to 16b.

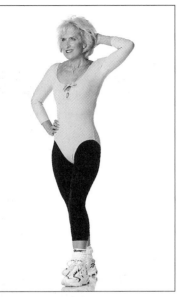
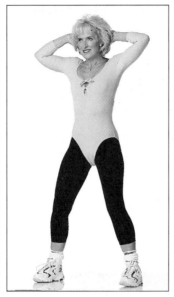
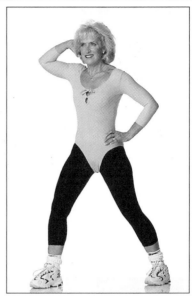
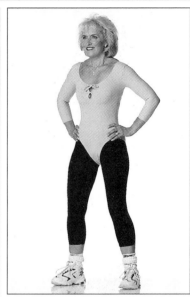

16b Half Jacks with Arms Start with your feet together, then tap the right toe out to the side, taking both arms out to the sides at the same time. Bring the feet together again and change to the other side. Keep changing from side to side for 8 repetitions, then move on to 16c.

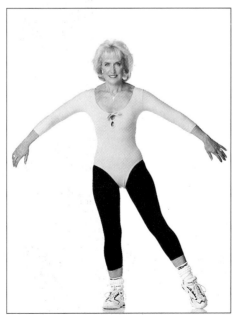

16c Double Scoops with Claps On the last half jack, turn to your right and make a scooping action with both arms as you lead off with the heel of the right foot, bringing the left foot close up behind. Immediately carry on with another scoop in the same direction, adding a clap, before turning back to repeat to the left. Repeat a double scoop to each side again before going back to the box step to repeat Sequence 3 again.

After completing each sequence twice through, go back to repeat each sequence once more to complete your 8 minutes.

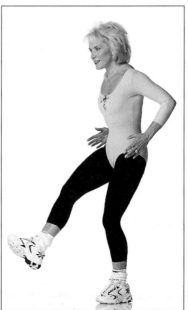
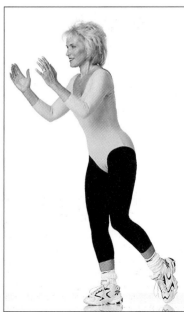

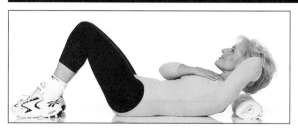

17 Abdominal Curl Lie on your back and place a towel under your head for comfort if you wish. Bend both knees, with your feet flat on the floor and your tummy pulled well in against the spine. Place one hand behind your head and the other hand across your chest. Now gently lift your head and shoulders off the floor, then lower again. Repeat 6 times slowly, breathing out as you lift and breathing in as you lower again. Rest and repeat.

18 Posture Improver Sit up, with your legs comfortably crossed. Keeping your head up and your back straight, place your hands on your shoulders. Now squeeze your shoulders back slowly and under control, then release. Repeat 4 times, then rest and do 4 more.

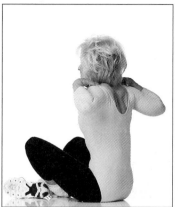

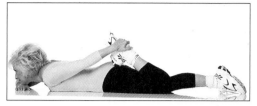

22 Front of Thigh Stretch Lie on your front, bend your right knee up and take hold of the ankle. Ease the heel close to the hip and push that hip firmly into the floor. Hold for 10 seconds, then change legs and repeat.

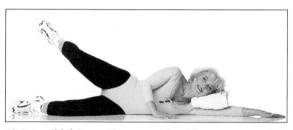

19 Outer Thigh Toner Lie on your side, with your arm extended and your head resting comfortably on a towel. Bend both legs so that each forms a 45-degree angle. Now lift the top leg to just above hip height, keeping the hips stacked on top of each other, then lower under control. Repeat 8 times, then change to the other leg and repeat.

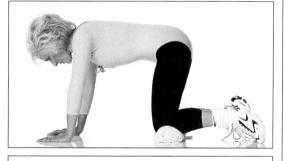

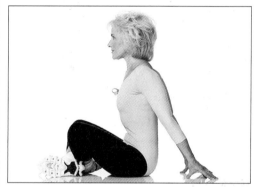

23 Chest Stretch Sit cross-legged and place your hands behind you on the floor. Now, sitting upright, squeeze the shoulders back to feel a stretch across the chest. Hold for 8 seconds, then release.

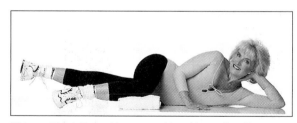

20 Inner Thigh Toner Lie on your side, with your head in your hand, or you can lie right down on your arm if it is more comfortable. Bring the top leg over the underneath leg and rest the knee on the towel. Now lift the underneath leg just off the floor, keeping the foot pulled towards you. Lift and lower under control 8 times, then change legs and repeat.

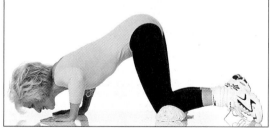

21 Press Ups Come up onto your hands and knees, with your hands under your shoulders and your knees under your hips. If you wish, you can place a towel under your knees to release any pressure. Now, keeping your tummy pulled in tight to protect the spine, slowly take your forehead down towards the floor in front of your hands, then press back up again without locking the elbows at the top. Repeat 4 times slowly, then rest and repeat.

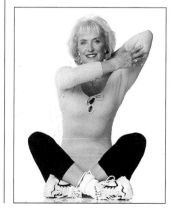

24 Underarm Stretch Sitting with legs crossed, head up and shoulders back, place your right hand behind your right shoulder and take the left hand across in front to push the arm further back. Hold for 6 seconds, then change sides and repeat.

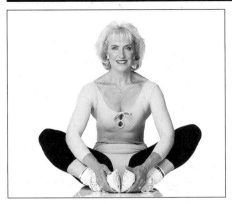

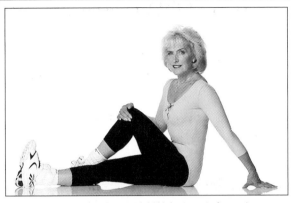

25 Inner Thigh Stretch Sit with soles of the feet together and your hands around your ankles. Now sit up tall and, with a straight back, lean forward slightly to place the elbows on the insides of the knees. Press down gently to feel a stretch on the insides of the thighs. Hold for 10 seconds, then try to press further to develop the stretch more. Hold for 5 more seconds, then release.

26 Outer Thigh Stretch Sit with both legs out in front, then cross your right leg over the left and place your right foot in line with the left knee. Now place your left hand on the outside of the right knee and the other hand on the floor for support. Gently squeeze the right knee further across the chest to feel a stretch in the outer thigh. Hold for 8 seconds, then release. Change legs and repeat.

27 Back of Thigh Stretch Lie on your back, with both knees bent and feet flat on the floor and take hold behind one knee. Now extend the held leg to feel the stretch in the back of the thigh. Keep your hips on the floor and move one hand further up the leg for support. Hold for 10 seconds, then try to extend the knee a little further in order to develop the stretch more. Hold for a further 10 seconds, then release and repeat with the other leg.

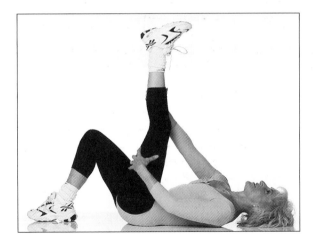

28 Full Body Stretch Lie on your back and take both arms over your head as you extend both legs away from you. Hold for 8 seconds, then slowly release.

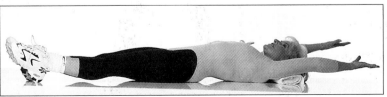

POSITIVE THOUGHT FOR THE DAY

I am often asked if exercise is essential to weight loss. Amazingly, the answer is no. Without doubt, it is what we eat that determines our weight, and calories do count. I never detail the calorie content in any of my diets because it isn't necessary. I've done all that for you, and if you follow any of my menus you should lose weight. The reduction of fat in the diet helps to minimise the fat on the body. The result is weight and inch loss, particularly from the areas we want to slim down.

So what about exercise? Exercise burns calories because of the extra energy we expend. It also works our muscles, and the bigger our muscles, the higher our metabolic rate. With exercise there is definitely a win-win situation. Aerobic exercise burns fat because, as we draw in more oxygen by forcing the heart to beat faster and the lungs to demand extra oxygen, this oxygen circulates in the bloodstream and combines with the carbohydrate stores in our muscles and also, very importantly, the fat that is stored around our muscles. The combination of the oxygen, glycogen (carbohydrate stores) and fat provides the energy we need to carry on exercising. This is why aerobic exercise is a fat-burning activity. Specific toning exercises make the muscles work harder. Unlike aerobic exercise where we use many muscles a little for quite a long time, toning exercises require much stronger work from the muscles because we are performing a concentrated number of repetitions and then allowing the muscles to rest before we repeat the exercise. Challenging the muscles in this way encourages them to become bigger and stronger, and the more muscle we have, the more calories we burn. So while it is possible to lose weight simply by restricting our calorie intake, we will enjoy even greater benefits if we expend additional calories through exercise, burn fat and work the muscles to give us a better shape.

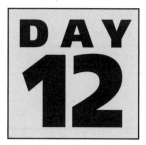

DAY 12

One of my slimmers wrote: 'My husband says I now have the figure I had when he married me 30 years ago'. Another lady wrote: 'My husband has regained his boyish figure again'. This diet will work just as effectively for men and women, no matter what their age.

Success in dieting is all about knowing that you will win. Most diets actually work, but few give such immediate results in real terms. I'm not interested in diets that claim you will 'lose 10lb in 10 days', because if you did, most of what you lost would be water and some would be muscle tissue. Only a little fat would burn away. As soon as you returned to 'normal eating' all the lost weight would almost certainly return. Such experiences only leave the dieter disappointed and disillusioned.

Now that you are well into your second week, your progress should be even faster. Not only are you more familiar with the exercises, but your body is also able to perform them in a more relaxed manner, thereby increasing their effectiveness. The daily workouts combine an aerobic workout that burns fat with muscle-toning exercises that give more definition to your body shape and strengthen your muscles and bones. Both types of exercise will help prevent the brittle bone disease osteoporosis. Our bones need to be challenged, and by working the muscles that are attached to them, bone strength and density is encouraged. This gives you an added incentive to make exercise part of your lifestyle, not just for this 28 days but also in the long term.

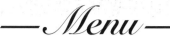

BREAKFAST

1 poached egg served on 1 slice of wholemeal toast

OR

2 bananas sliced and topped with 1 × 150g (5oz) raspberry diet yogurt

LUNCH

200g (7oz) baked beans served cold with a large salad of mixed vegetables and 2 teaspoons reduced-oil salad dressing, plus 1 × 150g (5oz) diet yogurt

OR

Jacket potato (approx. 225g/8oz) topped with 50g (2oz) chopped chicken, 25g (1oz) peas and 25g (1oz) sweetcorn mixed with 75g (3oz) plain diet yogurt flavoured with 1/2 a teaspoon of curry powder, plus a wedge of melon

DINNER

115g (4oz) lean steak, grilled and served with jacket potato (approx. 150g/5oz) and unlimited vegetables including boiled mushrooms and grilled tomatoes
PLUS
FRUITY APPLE TERRINE
(see recipe, page 177)

OR

LENTIL ROAST
(see recipe, page178)
PLUS
COEURS A LA CREME
(see recipe, page 176)

WARM UP – MOBILITY AND PULSE-RAISING

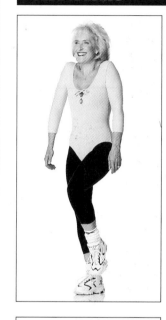

1 March on the Spot with Shoulder Lifts
Stand up straight, with your head up and your shoulders back, and march on the spot. As you march, lift both shoulders up towards your ears and then down again, keeping the action slow and controlled. Lift the shoulders for 2 marches and then lower them for 2 to keep a rhythmical pace. Lift and lower the shoulders 8 times altogether.

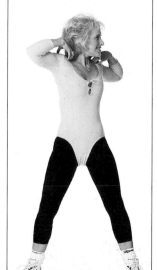

2 Waist Twists
Stand upright, with feet apart, tummy pulled in and knees slightly bent. Now place your hands on your shoulders and twist round as far as you can go, keeping the hips facing forward. Return to face front and do the same to the other side. Keep it smooth and controlled. Do 12, changing sides each time.

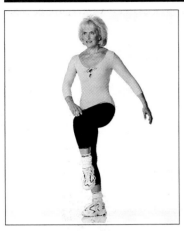

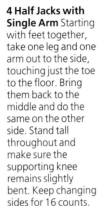

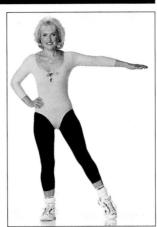

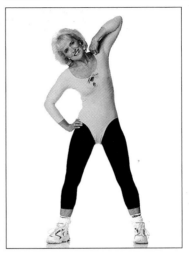

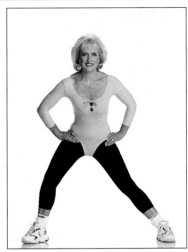

4 Half Jacks with Single Arm Starting with feet together, take one leg and one arm out to the side, touching just the toe to the floor. Bring them back to the middle and do the same on the other side. Stand tall throughout and make sure the supporting knee remains slightly bent. Keep changing sides for 16 counts.

3 Knee Lifts Take a step out to the side with the right leg then lift the left knee up to waist height, keeping your back straight and your head up. Try to touch the raised knee with the opposite hand. Perform 24, alternating legs.

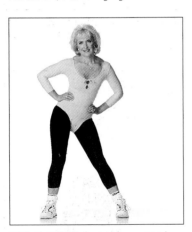

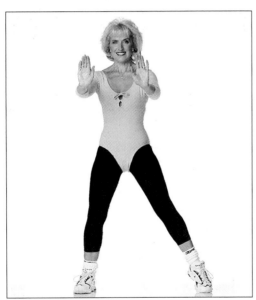

5 Hip Rolls With feet wide apart and knees bent, roll the hips around in a full circle, from the side, round to the front, and then to the back. Keep it very smooth and under control. Repeat 4 times slowly in one direction, then change direction and repeat.

6 Double Steps with Arm Presses Take 2 steps to the right and, at the same time, press both arms out in front at chest height. Now take 2 steps back to the left. Keep your body upright, with your shoulders back and your head up. Repeat the sequence 4 times altogether.

7 Waist Stretch Stand with feet apart, place your right hand on your shoulder and place your left hand at the top of your left thigh for support. Now gently lean to the left until you feel the right elbow is pointing up to the ceiling to feel a stretch down the waist. Hold for 6 seconds, then change sides and repeat.

8 Inner Thigh Stretch Take the legs very wide and place one foot out diagonally, with the knee bent in line with the toes. The other leg is straight, with the foot pointing forward. To feel the stretch on the inside of the thigh, take the straight leg further away from you. Hold for 6 seconds, then change legs and repeat.

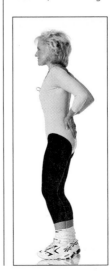

◀ **9 Chest Stretch** Stand with feet slightly apart and your head up. Now place your hands in the small of your back and squeeze your elbows back behind you to feel a stretch across the chest. Hold for 6 seconds, then release.

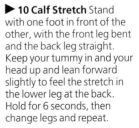

▶ **10 Calf Stretch** Stand with one foot in front of the other, with the front leg bent and the back leg straight. Keep your tummy in and your head up and lean forward slightly to feel the stretch in the lower leg at the back. Hold for 6 seconds, then change legs and repeat.

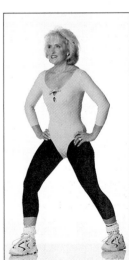

11 Back of Thigh Stretch

Stand with your back leg bent and your front leg straight, and place your hands in the middle of your thighs. Now, keeping your head up and your back flat, lean forward until you feel a stretch in the back of the straight leg. Hold for 6 seconds, then change legs and repeat.

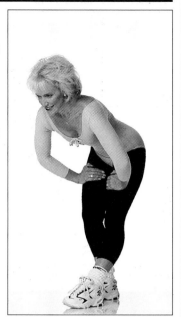

Today you are going to repeat each sequence twice through before moving to the next sequence. Once this is complete, go back to Sequence 1 and repeat each sequence once more, trying to add more energy to every move.

SEQUENCE 1

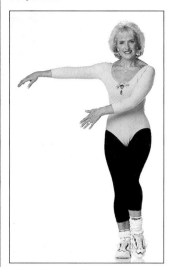
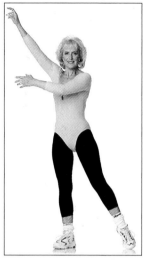
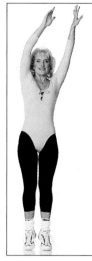
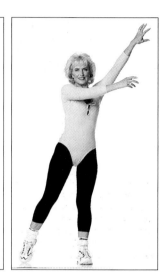

12 Front of Thigh Stretch

Take hold around one ankle so that the knee points towards the floor and the knees are fairly close together. Try to keep the knee of the supporting leg slightly bent and push the hip forward on the held leg to feel the stretch down the front of the thigh. Hold for 6 seconds, then change legs and repeat.

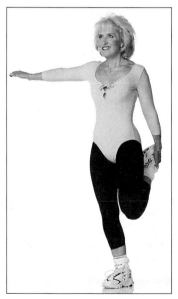

13a Step Touch Swing Step from side to side, swinging your arms to just above chest height. Make the steps wide and bend your knees well as you step out. Keep your head up and your back lifted. Repeat 8 times before moving on to 13b.

13b Travel Overs Now take 2 steps to the right, taking your arms over in a circular motion in front of you. Then take 2 steps to the left, letting your arms swing naturally over the top. Repeat twice through to each side then move on to 13c.

13c Touch Backs On the return from the final travel over take the right toe to touch the floor behind you and push the arms forward at the same time. Lean forward slightly to protect your back, and keep your tummy pulled in tight. Repeat 8 times before going back to the step touch swing to repeat Sequence 1 again.

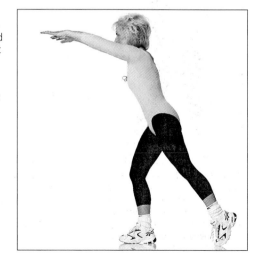

SEQUENCE 2

14a Hopscotch with Elbow Presses Step out to the side with the right leg and bend the left knee up behind you. At the same time your arms are up at chest height and the elbows press behind you as you lift the leg. Keep your body upright, tummy pulled in tightly and keep the knee of the supporting leg slightly bent. Do 8 hopscotches before changing to 14b.

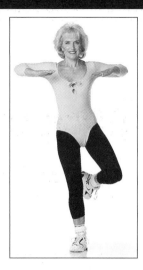

14b Walks with Rolling Arms Walk forward for 3 counts, stop on the 4th count and clap your hands. Now do the same thing but moving backwards. Try to roll your arms up at chest height as you walk. Repeat forward and back twice before moving on to 14c.

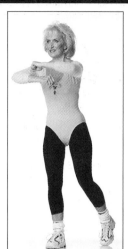

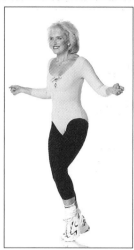

14c Skip Turns On the return from the last walk back, take a turn on the spot all the way round to your right, using a small bouncing skip. Make sure the heels land on the floor on each skip. (If you don't want to skip, you can march instead.) Use 4 counts to turn to the right then another 4 to turn to the left. Now go back to the hopscotch to repeat Sequence 2 again.

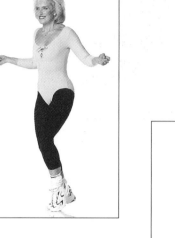

SEQUENCE 3

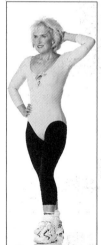
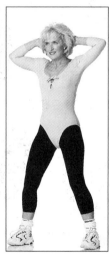
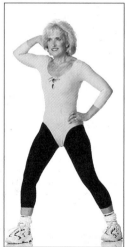
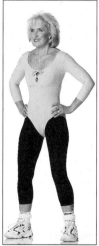
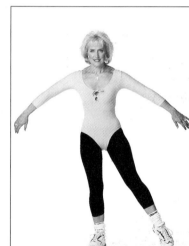
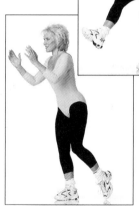

15a Box Step with Funky Arms Take one step forward and out with the right foot, placing your right hand at the side of your head at the same time. Now take the other foot forward, placing your left hand on your head. As you step back on the right, bring that hand back to the hip, then do the same on the left. Keep stepping forward and back rhythmically 4 times before changing to 15b.

15b Half Jacks with Arms Start with your feet together, then tap the right toe out to the side, taking both arms out to the sides at the same time. Bring the feet together again and change to the other side. Keep changing from side to side for 8 repetitions, then move on to 15c.

15c Double Scoops with Claps On the last half jack, turn to your right and make a scooping action with both arms as you lead off with the heel of the right foot, bringing the left foot close up behind. Immediately carry on with another scoop in the same direction, adding a clap, before turning back to repeat to the left. Repeat a double scoop to each side again before going back to the box step to repeat Sequence 3 again.

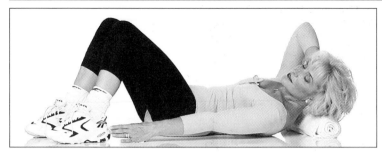

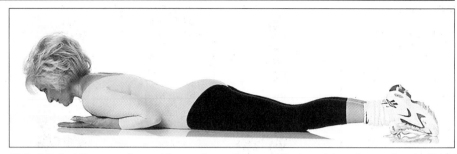

16 Waist Reach Lie on your back, with your knees bent and feet flat on the floor. Place a rolled towel under your head and place your right hand behind your head. Use your left hand to reach round towards your left ankle, with your head slightly raised. Come back to the centre and swap hands to reach down the other side. Keep your tummy pulled in tight against your spine and keep the movement slow and controlled. Repeat 4 times to each side, then rest and repeat.

17 Back Raises Lie on your front, with your elbows close to your waist and the palms up. Keep looking at the floor as you slowly lift the upper body about 7.5cm (3in) from the floor, and lower again. Keep both feet firmly on the floor. Repeat 4 times, breathing out as you lift and breathing in as you lower. Rest and repeat.

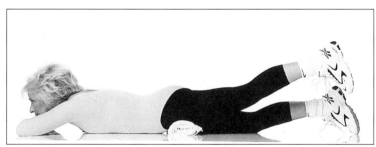

▶ **19 Press Ups** Come up onto your hands and knees, with your hands under your shoulders and your knees under your hips. If you wish, you can place a towel under your knees to release any pressure. Now, keeping your tummy pulled in tight to protect the spine, slowly take your forehead down towards the floor in front of your hands, then press back up again without locking the elbows at the top. Repeat 4 times slowly, then rest and repeat.

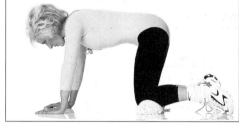

▼ **20 Inner Thigh Toner** Lie on your side, with your head in your hand, or you can lie right down on your arm if it is more comfortable. Bring the top leg over the underneath leg and rest the knee on the towel. Now lift the underneath leg just off the floor, keeping the foot pulled towards you. Lift and lower under control 8 times, then change legs and repeat.

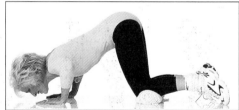

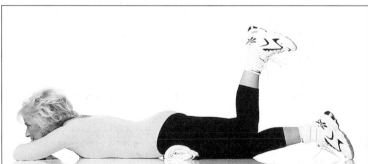

18 Bottom and Back of Thigh Toner Lie on your front, with your head resting on your hands, your upper body relaxed and the towel under your hips. Now lift one leg off the floor, keeping the hips facing the floor, then bend the knee and bring the heel towards the hip to work the back of the thigh. Straighten again, then lower the whole leg back to the floor. Repeat 4 times, then repeat on the other leg.

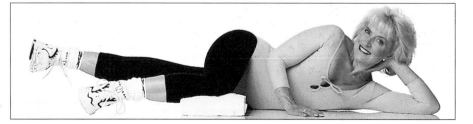

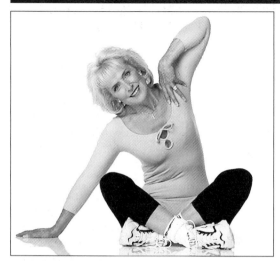

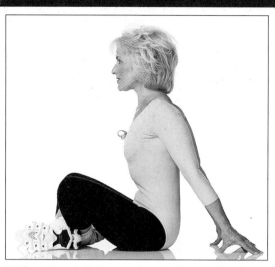

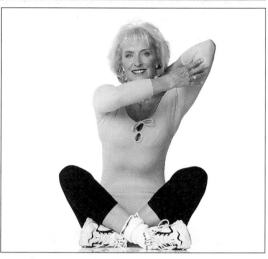

22 Waist Stretch Sit comfortably cross-legged, with your back straight and your head up. Now place your right hand on your right shoulder and place your left hand on the floor for support. Bend over to the side toward the hand on the floor, lifting the right elbow up toward the ceiling. Keep the hips securely on the floor and try not to lean forward or back. Hold for 6 seconds, then change sides and repeat.

23 Chest Stretch Sitting cross-legged, place your hands behind you on the floor. Now, sitting upright, squeeze the shoulders back to feel a stretch across the chest. Hold for 8 seconds, then release.

24 Underarm Stretch Sitting with legs crossed, head up and shoulders back, place your right hand behind your right shoulder and take the left hand across in front to push the arm further back. Hold for 6 seconds, then change sides and repeat.

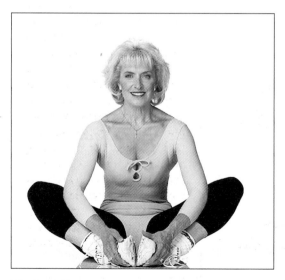

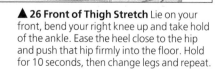

◀ **25 Inner Thigh Stretch** Sit with the soles of the feet together and your hands around your ankles. Now sit up tall and, with a straight back, lean forward slightly to place the elbows on the insides of the knees. Press down gently to feel a stretch on the insides of the thighs. Hold for 10 seconds, then try to press further to develop the stretch more. Hold for 5 more seconds, then release.

▲ **26 Front of Thigh Stretch** Lie on your front, bend your right knee up and take hold of the ankle. Ease the heel close to the hip and push that hip firmly into the floor. Hold for 10 seconds, then change legs and repeat.

27a Bottom Stretch Lie on your back, with both knees bent and feet flat on the floor. Draw one knee into the chest, holding underneath the knee, and squeeze the raised leg towards the chest to feel a stretch in your bottom. Hold for 10 seconds, then move on to 27b.

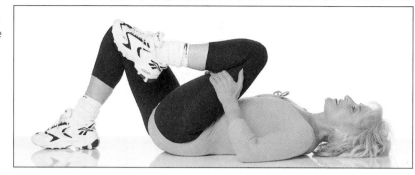

27b Back of Thigh Stretch Now extend the leg further to feel the stretch move to the back of the thigh. Keep your hips on the floor and move one hand further up the leg for support. Hold for 10 seconds, then try to extend the knee a little further in order to develop the stretch more. Hold for a further 10 seconds, then release.

Repeat 27a and 27b on the other leg.

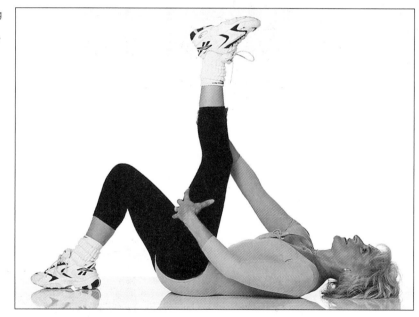

28 Full Body Stretch Lie on your back and take both arms over your head as you extend both legs away from you. Hold for 8 seconds, then slowly release.

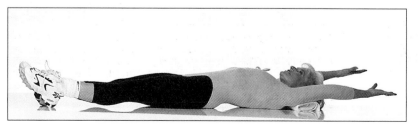

POSITIVE THOUGHT FOR THE DAY

In today's introduction I referred to the importance of exercise in your weight-loss campaign. Exercise is vital if you are to continue to lose weight and inches at a satisfactory rate and it will also help you maintain your new figure so that you do not return to your previous shape.

The metabolic rate is the rate at which we burn energy. We should always consume sufficient calories to keep the metabolism buoyant. There is little danger of it slowing down too much if we eat around 1,400 calories a day. Added to this is the discovery of the effect on the body of fat calories compared with carbohydrate calories. Research has shown that the body burns carbohydrate easily but unfortunately stores the fat that we eat. This is why low-fat diets work so efficiently. You can eat plenty of carbohydrates to satisfy your appetite. That's why so many followers of my diets have said that the most important contributory factor to their success was the large amount of food they were allowed to eat. How can anyone seriously stick to a diet if they are hungry? The freedom to eat as many vegetables as you want at mealtimes resolves this problem.

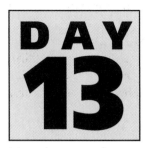

DAY 13

As you approach the end of your second week don't even think about cheating! Just having a little treat here or there can add up sufficiently to stop the diet from working. More importantly, once we start nibbling at things our willpower slides down a very slippery slope. One biscuit becomes a whole packet, one chocolate bar turns into three and, before we know where we are, we've trapped ourselves into a wholesale binge. I'm not saying you'll never binge again, but please don't do it today. I want you to reach the beginning of Day 15 and the next weighing and measuring session without having faltered seriously.

Take another rest day from the formal exercises today, but try to stay as active as possible in your daily activities. Avoid temptation by doing something outside the kitchen. Now is not the time to start baking cakes for your freezer!

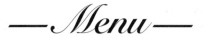

—Menu—

BREAKFAST

1 fresh crusty bread roll (approx. 50g/2oz) spread with 2 teaspoons of marmalade or honey

OR

25g (1oz) very lean bacon, grilled and served with 115g (4oz) mushrooms cooked in vegetable stock, 75g (3oz) baked beans and 200g (7oz) tinned tomatoes

LUNCH

115g (4oz) boiled brown rice (cooked weight) mixed with 25g (1oz) each of peas, sweetcorn, red and green peppers, cucumber, a few spring onions and 1 chopped tomato, plus a low-fat fromage frais or diet yogurt

OR

4 Ryvitas or 40g (1½oz) wholemeal bread spread with reduced-oil salad dressing or a little horseradish sauce and 75g (3oz) salmon, tuna (in brine) or mackerel, topped with sliced cucumber, plus 1 piece of fresh fruit

DINNER

225g (8oz) white fish, steamed, microwaved or grilled and served with steamed sliced mushrooms, 150g (5oz) mashed potatoes, unlimited vegetables and tomato sauce if desired
PLUS
STRAWBERRY WINE JELLY
(see recipe, page 183)

OR

RATATOUILLE
(see recipe, page 181) served with 150g (5oz) potatoes and unlimited vegetables
PLUS
RASPBERRY AND STRAWBERRY BAVAROIS
(see recipe, page 181)

POSITIVE THOUGHT FOR THE DAY

When I am trying to be stricter than usual with myself, I plan a really busy week so that I am out more than is customary. Many slimmers make this an excuse for not sticking to the diet, but I find it much easier if I'm away from the kitchen and the kettle! All those cups of tea do add up, and the fridge is always there ready to beckon when a hunger pang lingers. If we keep our minds busy we can consciously ignore our tummies, which often only tell us we're hungry because we're bored. We then end up eating for entertainment rather than nourishment. It is a habit we should try to curb.

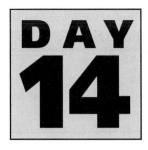

DAY 14

It's the last day of Week 2 and I suggest that you have your main meal at lunchtime again to allow more time for you to work it off before tomorrow's assessment.

You will notice that I never include rice and pasta in the menus on the last day of the week to avoid causing an artificial weight gain – the last thing you want for tomorrow morning. Alcohol has a dehydrating effect and results in excessive thirst, so don't have more than your usual one drink tonight. If on any occasion you wake up in the night gasping for water, think back to the meal you had and recognise which recipes make you thirsty. Avoid these in future, or cut down on the seasoning. Work hard at your exercises today and be as active as possible. Have a good day!

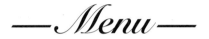

—Menu—

BREAKFAST

50g (2oz) Kellogg's All-Bran with milk from allowance and 2 teaspoons of sugar

OR

1 slice of wholemeal toast with 2 teaspoons marmalade or honey, plus either 1 small banana or 115g (4oz) strawberries

LUNCH

115g (4oz) chicken (no skin) served with unlimited vegetables including 115g (4oz) potatoes
PLUS
2 pieces of fresh fruit or 1 Marks & Spencer Lite Mousse

OR

1 egg omelette cooked in a non-stick pan and stuffed with 50g (2oz) low-fat fromage frais mixed with sliced boiled mushrooms and chopped green peppers and served with a large salad
PLUS
PINEAPPLE AND ORANGE SORBET
(see recipe, page 180)

SUPPER

Seafood salad (using seafood of your choice, e.g seafood sticks, crab, prawns etc. to make a total weight of 150g/5oz) served on a mixed green salad topped with SEAFOOD DRESSING (see recipe, page 182), plus ¹/₂ a honeydew melon, seeded, chopped and topped with 1 × 150g (5oz) diet yogurt, any flavour
OR
Quorn burger served with unlimited vegetables excluding potatoes, plus 1 × 150g (5oz) diet yogurt mixed with 115g (4oz) fresh fruit of your choice

1 Knee Bends with Wide Arms

Stand with legs wide apart and feet turned out slightly. Now bend your knees in line with the toes, taking your hips back as if you were trying to sit in a chair. At the same time, bring both arms out to the sides to shoulder height. Come up without locking the knees fully, bringing your arms down by your sides. Repeat 8 times slowly.

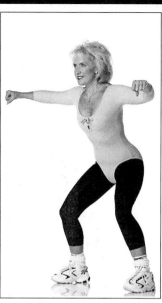

2 Step Touch with Bicep Curls

Stand tall and step out to alternate sides, bending your knees as the feet come together. At the same time bend alternate elbows, keeping them close to the waist. Perform 16 times altogether.

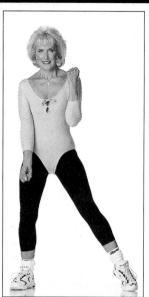
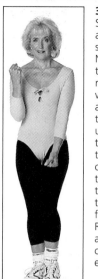

3 Side Bends

Stand with feet apart and knees slightly bent. Now lean over to the right side, reaching out with the right arm and lifting the left elbow up. Come up to the centre and then lean to the other side. Keep the hips still throughout and try not to lean forward or back. Repeat 12 times altogether, changing sides each time.

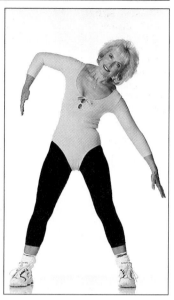

4 Neck Mobiliser

Stand with feet apart, tummy in and shoulders back. Now slowly turn your head to the right, keeping the shoulders facing front. Return to the centre and repeat to the other side. Repeat only 3 times to each side.

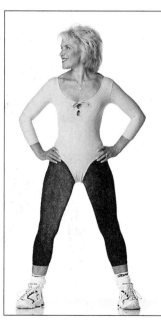

5 Double Steps with Arm Presses

Take 2 steps to the right and, at the same time, press both arms out in front at chest height. Now take 2 steps back to the left. Keep your body upright, with your shoulders back and your head up. Repeat the sequence 4 times altogether.

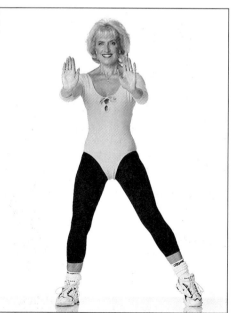

6 Hip Rolls

With feet wide apart and knees bent, roll the hips around in a full circle, from the side, round to the front, and then to the back. Keep it very smooth and under control. Repeat 4 times slowly in one direction, then change direction and repeat.

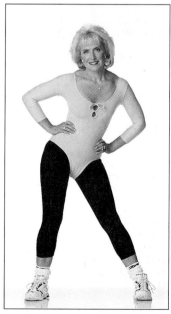

7 Chest Stretch
Stand with feet slightly apart and your head up. Now place your hands in the small of your back and squeeze your elbows back behind you to feel a stretch across the chest. Hold for 6 seconds, then release.

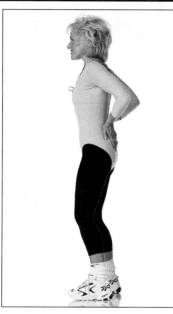

8 Upper Back Stretch
Standing with feet comfortably apart, bring your arms round in front of your chest and clasp your hands together. Drop your head forward and gently press the arms away from the hands to feel a stretch across the shoulder blades at the back. Hold for 6 seconds, then release.

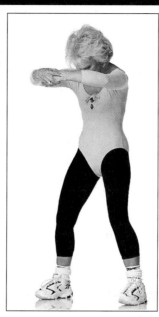

9 Inner Thigh Stretch Take the legs very wide and place one foot out diagonally, with the knee bent in line with the toes. The other leg is straight, with the foot pointing forward. To feel the stretch on the inside of the thigh, take the straight leg further away from you. Hold for 6 seconds, then change legs and repeat.

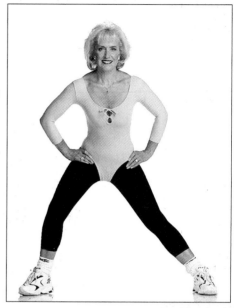

10 Front of Thigh Stretch
Take hold around one ankle so that the knee points toward the floor and the knees are fairly close together. Try to keep the knee of the supporting leg slightly bent and push the hip forward on the held leg to feel the stretch down the front of the thigh. Hold for 6 seconds, then change legs and repeat.

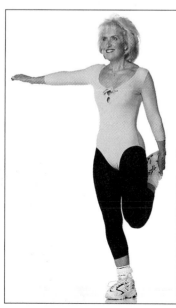

11 Back of Thigh Stretch
Stand with your back leg bent and your front leg straight, and place your hands in the middle of your thighs. Now, keeping your head up and your back flat, lean forward until you feel a stretch in the back of the straight leg. Hold for 6 seconds, then change legs and repeat.

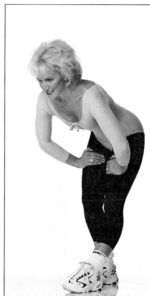

12 Calf Stretch
Stand with one foot in front of the other, with the front leg bent and the back leg straight. Keep your tummy in and your head up and lean forward slightly to feel the stretch in the lower leg at the back. Hold for 6 seconds, then change legs and repeat.

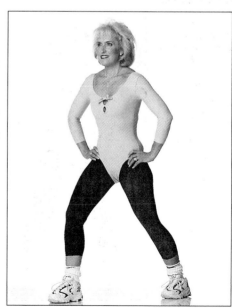

SEQUENCE 1

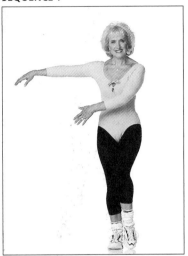
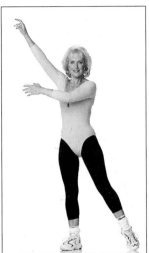
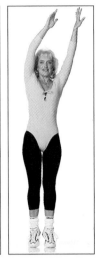
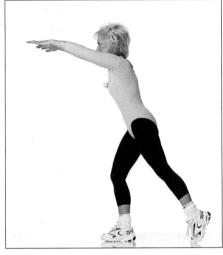
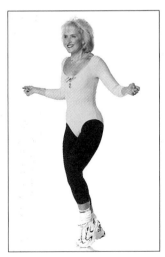

13a Step Touch Swing Step from side to side, swinging your arms to just above chest height. Make the steps wide and bend your knees well as you step out. Keep your head up and your back lifted. Repeat 8 times before moving on to 13b.

13b Travel Overs Now take 2 steps to the right, taking your arms over in a circular motion in front of you. Then take 2 steps to the left, letting your arms swing naturally over the top. Repeat twice through to each side then move on to 13c.

13c Touch Backs On the return from the final travel over take the right toe to touch the floor behind you and push the arms forward at the same time. Lean forward slightly to protect your back, and keep your tummy pulled in tight. Repeat 8 times before going back to the step touch swing to repeat Sequence 1 again.

SEQUENCE 2

14a Hopscotch with Elbow Presses Step out to the side with the right leg and bend the left knee up behind you. At the same time your arms are up at chest height and the elbows press behind you as you lift the leg. Keep your body upright, tummy pulled in tightly and keep the knee of the supporting leg slightly bent. Do 8 hopscotches before changing to 14b.

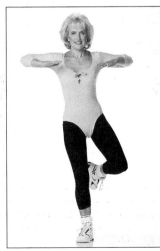

14b Walks with Rolling Arms Walk forward for 3 counts, stop on the 4th count and clap your hands. Now do the same thing but moving backwards. Try to roll your arms up at chest height as you walk. Repeat forward and back twice before moving on to 14c.

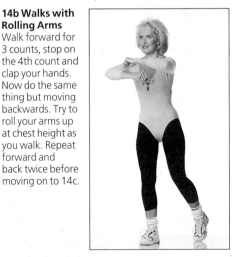

14c Skip Turns On the return from the last walk back, take a turn on the spot all the way round to your right, using a small bouncing skip. Make sure the heels land on the floor on each skip. (If you don't want to skip, you can march instead.) Use 4 counts to turn to the right then another 4 to turn to the left. Now go back to the hopscotch to repeat Sequence 2 again.

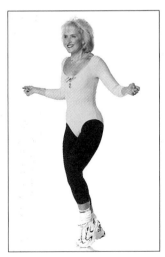

SEQUENCE 3

15a Box Step with Funky Arms Take one step forward and out with the right foot, placing your right hand at the side of your head at the same time. Now take the other foot forward, placing your left hand on your head. As you step back on the right, bring that hand back to the hip, then do the same on the left. Keep stepping forward and back rhythmically 4 times before changing to 15b.

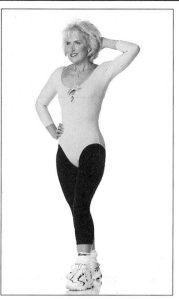 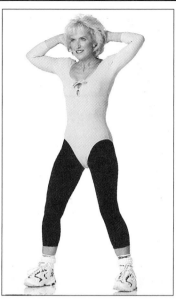 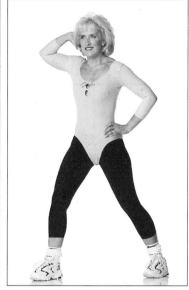 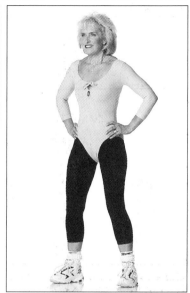

15b Half Jacks with Arms Start with your feet together, then tap the right toe out to the side, taking both arms out to the sides at the same time. Bring the feet together again and change to the other side. Keep changing from side to side for 8 repetitions, then move on to 15c.

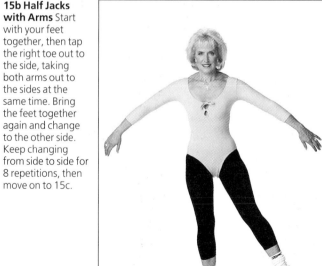

15c Double Scoops with Claps On the last half jack, turn to your right and make a scooping action with both arms as you lead off with the heel of the right foot, bringing the left foot close up behind. Immediately carry on with another scoop in the same direction, adding a clap, before turning back to repeat to the left. Repeat a double scoop to each side again before going back to the box step to repeat Sequence 3 again.

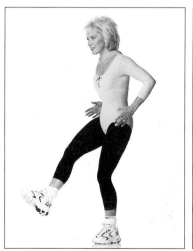 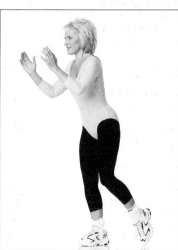

Repeat each sequence twice through before moving to the next sequence, then go back to Sequence 1 and repeat each sequence once more, trying to add more energy to every move.

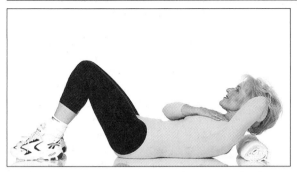

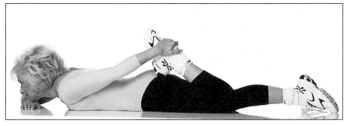

16 Abdominal Curl Lie on your back and place a towel under your head for comfort if you wish. Bend both knees, with your feet flat on the floor and your tummy pulled well in against the spine. Place one hand behind your head and the other hand across your chest. Now gently lift your head and shoulders off the floor, then lower again. Repeat 6 times slowly, breathing out as you lift and breathing in as you lower again. Rest and repeat.

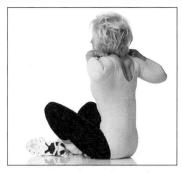

17 Posture Improver Sit up, with your legs comfortably crossed. Keeping your head up and your back straight, place your hands on your shoulders. Now squeeze your shoulders back slowly and under control, then release. Repeat 4 times, then rest and do 4 more.

18 Outer Thigh Toner Lie on your side, with your arm extended and your head resting comfortably on a towel. Bend both legs so that each forms a 45-degree angle. Now lift the top leg to just above hip height, keeping the hips stacked on top of each other, then lower under control. Repeat 8 times, then change to the other leg.

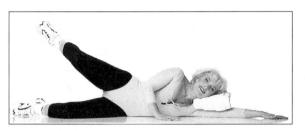

19 Bottom and Back of Thigh Toner Lie on your front, with your head resting on your hands, your upper body relaxed and the towel under your hips. Now lift one leg off the floor, keeping the hips facing the floor, then bend the knee and bring the heel toward the hip to work the back of the thigh. Straighten again, then lower the whole leg back to the floor. Repeat 4 times, then repeat on the other leg.

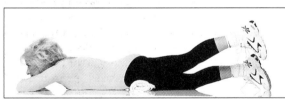

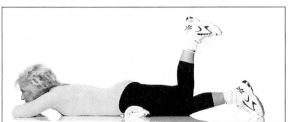

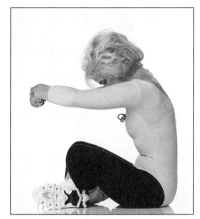

20 Front of Thigh Stretch Lie on your front, bend your right knee up and take hold of the ankle. Ease the heel close to the hip and push that hip firmly into the floor. Hold for 10 seconds, then change legs and repeat.

21 Upper Back Stretch Sit cross-legged, bring both arms round in front of you at chest height and clasp your hands. Drop your head forward, and round your spine to feel a stretch across the back of the shoulders. Hold for 8 seconds, then release.

22 Inner Thigh Stretch Sit with soles of the feet together and your hands around your ankles. Now sit up tall and, with a straight back, lean forward slightly to place the elbows on the insides of the knees. Press down gently to feel a stretch on the insides of the thighs. Hold for 10 seconds, then try to press further to develop the stretch more. Hold for 5 more seconds, then release.

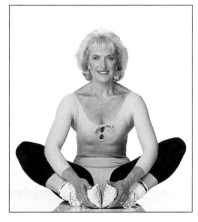

23 Outer Thigh Stretch Sit with both legs out in front, then cross your right leg over the left and place your right foot in line with the left knee. Now place your left hand on the outside of the right knee and the other hand on the floor for support. Gently squeeze the right knee further across the chest to feel a stretch in the outer thigh. Hold for 8 seconds, then release. Change legs and repeat.

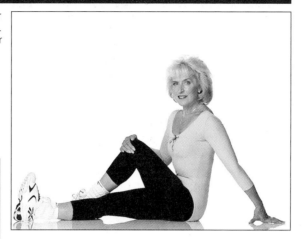

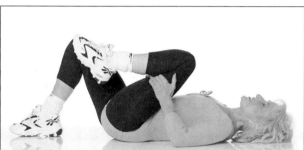

24a Bottom Stretch Lie on your back, with both knees bent and feet flat on the floor. Draw one knee into your chest, holding underneath the knee, and squeeze the raised leg towards the chest to feel a stretch in your bottom. Hold for 10 seconds, then move on to 24b.

24b Back of Thigh Stretch Now extend the leg further to feel the stretch move to the back of the thigh. Keep your hips on the floor and move one hand further up the leg for support. Hold for 10 seconds, then try to extend the knee a little further in order to develop the stretch more. Hold for a further 10 seconds, then release.

Repeat 24a and 24b on the other leg.

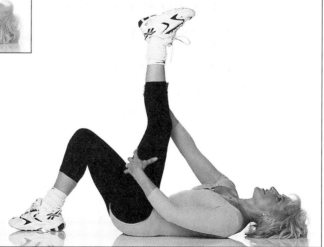

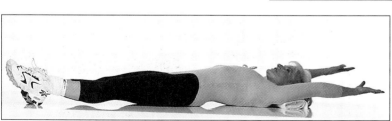

25 Full Body Stretch Lie on your back and take both arms over your head as you extend both legs away from you. Hold for 8 seconds, then slowly release.

POSITIVE THOUGHT FOR THE DAY

Cast your mind back to Day 1 of this programme and remember how unfit you felt and unsure of your ability to perform the exercises for the first time. Now, 14 days into the programme, your body is totally familiar with the tasks that have been set, your muscles have grown stronger, your body is leaner and there is less of you! You should be justly proud of your achievement so far, and I am sure you are looking forward to feeling even more full of energy at the end of the 28 days. The rest days are important because they enable your glycogen stores (that's the energy stores of carbohydrate in your muscles) to replenish completely. By challenging your muscles and your body through exercise and then allowing it time to rest and recover, you will develop a higher level of fitness and avoid any damage.

As this is your last day before your next weighing and measuring session, fill up on low-calorie drinks and enjoy your evening snack. Treat yourself to a special evening of entertainment – whether it be hiring a video you've been meaning to watch, going to the cinema or theatre, or just visiting a friend. Do keep yourself busy so you're not tempted to cheat. Attack temptation with activity and look forward to your second weighing and measuring day tomorrow. Best of luck!

DAY 15

After you've visited the bathroom first thing this morning, find your tape measure and make a note of your latest inch loss progress. Now weigh yourself. Always use the same set of scales and, ideally, place them on a piece of wood or chipboard for a more accurate reading.

I have no doubt that you will have lost both inches and weight. However, as your muscle tone increases and your level of fat decreases, sometimes little registers on the scales. But the most important factor is that you like what you now see in the mirror better than two weeks ago.

The duration of your workout is extended this week to increase your rate of fat burning through your aerobic activity. You will realise how much fitter you have become in just 2 weeks. It's a great feeling.

So onward to Week 3. You are now halfway towards real success.

WEEK 3: TIME: 25 MINUTES			
5	**12**	**5**	**3**
WARM UP	AEROBIC	TONE	STRETCH

—Menu—

BREAKFAST

25g (1oz) muesli mixed with 150g (5oz) diet yogurt or 75g (3oz) low-fat fromage frais plus 1 sliced banana

OR

2 turkey rashers, dry-fried or grilled, plus 2 tomatoes and 115g (4oz) baked beans on 15g (½oz) toast

LUNCH

TRIPLE DECKER SANDWICH
(see recipe, page 184)
plus 1 × 150g (5oz) diet yogurt

OR

Jacket potato (approx. 225g/8oz) topped with 200g (7oz) baked beans, plus 225g (8oz) plums or similar fruit

DINNER

Barbecued pork kebabs (see recipe for BARBECUED CHICKEN KEBABS on page 174, and substitute pork steak for chicken). Serve with soy sauce and 150g (5oz) boiled brown rice (cooked weight per person) mixed with beansprouts
PLUS
APRICOT PLUM SOFTIE (see recipe, page 173)

OR

VEGETARIAN SPAGHETTI BOLOGNESE
(see recipe, page 185)
PLUS
115g (4oz) fruit sorbet

Plus an extra glass of wine to celebrate the successful completion of your second week.

WARM UP – MOBILITY AND PULSE-RAISING

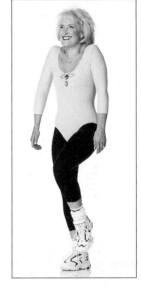

This week the warm-up session stays the same length of time, but now you are becoming fitter you should be able to work harder with each move to ensure it is more thorough and effective.

1 March on the Spot with Shoulder Lifts Stand up straight, with your head up and your shoulders back, and march on the spot. As you march, lift both shoulders up towards your ears and then down again, keeping the action slow and controlled. Lift the shoulders for 2 marches and then lower them for 2 to keep a rhythmical pace. Lift and lower the shoulders 8 times altogether.

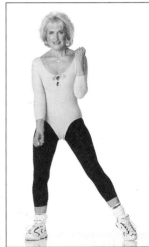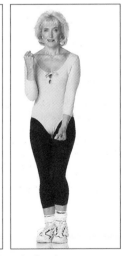

2 Step Touch with Bicep Curls Stand tall and step out to alternate sides, bending your knees as the feet come together. At the same time bend alternate elbows, keeping them close to the waist. Perform 16 times altogether.

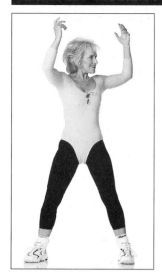

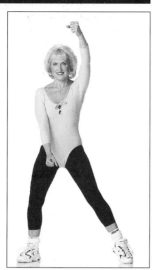

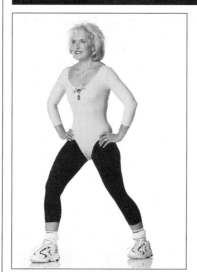

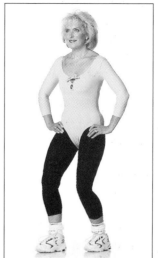

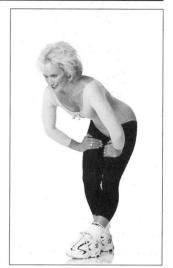

3 Waist Twists Stand with feet apart, tummy pulled in tight and knees slightly bent. Bring your arms up to shoulder height as shown then twist to alternate sides from the waist, keeping your hips still. Do 8 repetitions slowly and under control.

5 Squats with Arms With feet apart, bend from the knees, letting your hips dip back as if you were trying to sit in a chair. At the same time, draw your arms straight up in front of you to shoulder height. Look straight ahead, keeping your back flat and your tummy pulled in tight against your spine. Do 8 altogether.

4 Side Steps with Monkey Arms Take 2 steps out to the right, with your arms straight out in front, pulling them up and down alternately in rhythm with the steps. Take 2 steps back to the left and keep going, to repeat the sequence 4 times altogether.

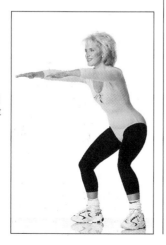

6 Calf Stretch Stand upright, with one foot in front of the other. Keep the back leg straight and bend the front leg and make sure both feet point forward. Lean towards the front leg to feel a stretch in the lower leg at the back. Now try to take the back leg further back to gain a more effective stretch. Hold for 8 seconds, then change legs and repeat.

9 Front of Thigh Stretch Take hold around one ankle so that the knee points towards the floor and the knees are fairly close together. Try to keep the knee of the supporting leg slightly bent and push the hip forward on the held leg to feel the stretch down the front of the thigh. Hold for 6 seconds, then change legs and repeat.

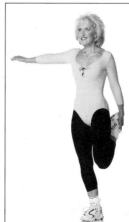

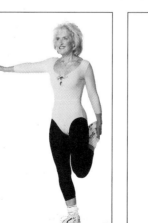

7 Lower Calf Stretch Now bring the back leg one step in towards the front leg and bend both knees, as if you were sitting on a stool. You should now feel the stretch further down the calf. Keep your head up and your back straight throughout. Hold for 6 seconds, then change legs and repeat.

8 Back of Thigh Stretch Keep the back leg bent, straighten the front leg and place your hands on the tops of your thighs. Lean forward, keeping your back flat and your head in line with your spine. To feel a greater stretch in the back of the thigh, lift the hips up more now. Hold for 8 seconds, then change legs and repeat.

10 Chest Stretch Stand with feet apart and knees slightly bent. Take both hands behind you and clasp them loosely together. Keeping the elbows bent, pull your shoulder blades back to feel a stretch across the chest. Make sure your head is up and your tummy is pulled in throughout. Hold for 6 seconds, then release.

WARM-UP STRETCH

11 Tricep Stretch Still standing with feet apart, tummy pulled in tight and knees slightly bent, take your right hand behind the right shoulder and use the left hand on the fleshy part of the right underarm to push it further back. Keep your head up throughout and hold for 6 seconds. Change arms and repeat.

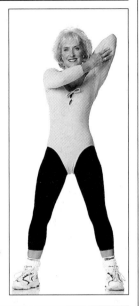

▼ 12 Inner Thigh Stretch Take the legs very wide and place one foot out diagonally, with the knee bent in line with the toes. The other leg is straight, with the foot pointing forward. To feel the stretch on the inside of the thigh, take the straight leg further away from you. Hold for 8 seconds, then change legs and repeat.

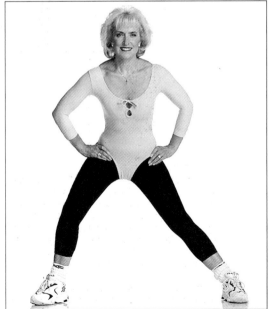

AEROBICS

This week, the length of time for this session has now increased to 12 minutes. You can gradually build up to this time throughout the week if you prefer. On Day 18 a whole new sequence is added to challenge you further and keep you coming back for more! Most of the moves will now be familiar to you, so you can probably move from one sequence straight on to the next without repeating, and then simply keep performing each sequence in turn until the time is complete. The first 2 minutes of this session should be fairly easy – you could perhaps leave out the arm movements. Then try to work hard in the middle for 8 minutes then let the intensity drop again for the last 2 minutes. This is a safe and effective way of performing aerobic, fat-burning moves because it allows the pulse rate to rise and fall safely.

SEQUENCE 1

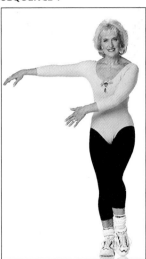 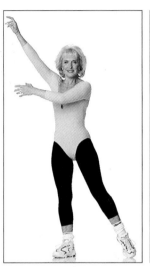 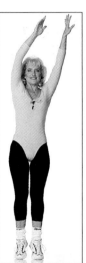 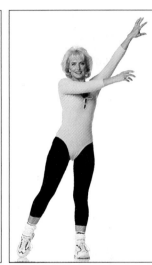

13a Step Touch Swing Step from side to side swinging the arms to just above shoulder height. Try to take wider steps now, with a deeper bend of the knees, but make sure you control the move and keep your head up and back straight. Repeat 8 times before moving on to 13b.

▲ 13b Travel Overs Take the 2 steps to the side, swinging your arms over in the direction that you are moving. You should now be able to add a small jump as the feet come together in the middle, but make sure your heels land on the floor if you add this. Repeat twice to each side before moving on to 13c.

13c Touch Backs As you come back from the final travel over, take the right leg back to touch the floor with the toe, leaning forward slightly and pushing your arms out in front at the same time. Do 8 touch backs with alternate legs before moving on to Sequence 2.

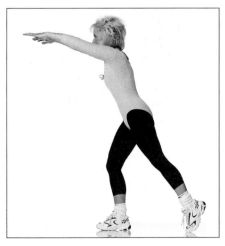

SEQUENCE 2

14a Hopscotch with Elbow Presses Take a step out to the side on the right leg and bend the left leg up behind. At the same time have your elbows up at shoulder height and, as the leg lifts at the back, press the elbows behind you, then repeat to the other side. Now make the steps wider and use the arms more strongly to make the move more effective. Do 8 times to alternate sides, then change to 14b.

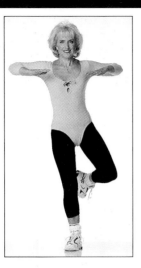

14b Walks with Rolling Arms Take 3 steps forward then clap, bringing the feet together on the 4th count, then take 3 steps back again. Roll the arms at chest height as you walk and now try to cover a lot more floor and keep tall. Repeat forward and back twice before moving on to 14c.

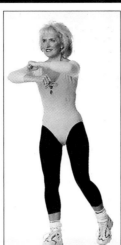

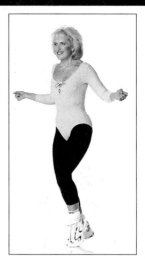

14c Skip Turns Take 4 counts to turn all the way round with a light skip, then go round the other way. Make sure the heels make contact with the floor and keep the trunk upright. Now move on to Sequence 3.

SEQUENCE 3

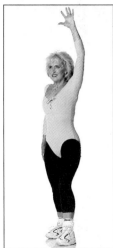

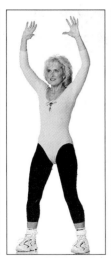

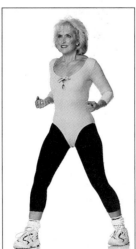

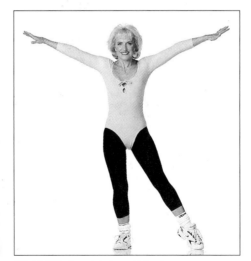

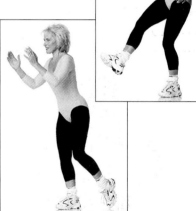

15a Box Step with High Arms Take a step forward with the right leg, leading with the heel, with the right arm overhead. Now do the same on the left side. This time, as you step back with alternate legs draw your elbows behind you at waist height with 2 little pushes. Step wide and use the arms strongly but keep your body upright. Do 4 box steps before moving on to 15b.

15b Half Jacks with Arms Take alternate toes out to the sides, bringing your arms out to just above shoulder height at the same time. As you change from one foot to the other add a small spring to increase the intensity of the move. Repeat 8 times under control before moving on to 15c.

15c Double Scoops with Claps On the last half jack, turn to your right and make a scooping action with both arms as you lead off with the heel of the right foot, bringing the left foot close up behind you. Take another scoop to the right, adding a clap at the end before turning to go left. Repeat a double scoop to each side again before starting again from Sequence 1.

Keep repeating the sequences from 1–3 until you feel you have done enough to challenge yourself.

As at the start of Week 2, there are changes to the exercises here, some of which you may be ready for and some you may not. You simply need to work to a point of discomfort if they are to be effective. However, we all progress at different rates, so do only as much as you are able to do and then rest.

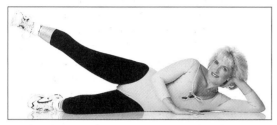

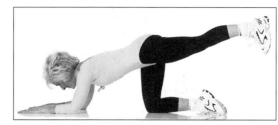

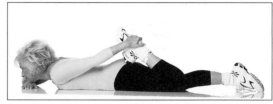

16 Outer Thigh Toner Lie on your side, propped on your elbow (or you can continue to use a towel if you prefer). The underneath leg is bent and the top leg is now straight, with the hips stacked on top of each other. Now lift the top leg to just above hip height, keeping the foot pointing forward and without tipping the hips back. Lower the leg again and repeat. Do 12 repetitions, then rest and repeat. Roll over and repeat with the other leg.

18 Bottom Toner Come up onto your forearms and knees, and place a towel under the knees if it helps. Pull your tummy in tightly and extend one leg out behind you with the toe on the floor. Now lift the leg under control to just above hip height and then lower it again. Keep both hips facing the floor and take care not to swing the leg. Do 12 repetitions, then change legs and repeat.

21 Front of Thigh Stretch Lie on your front, bend your right knee up and take hold of the ankle. Ease the heel close to the hip and push that hip firmly into the floor. Hold for 10 seconds, then change legs and repeat.

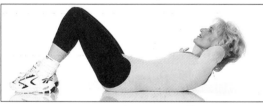

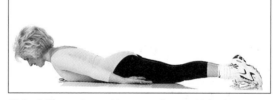

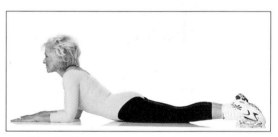

17 Abdominal Curl Lie on your back, with your knees bent and your feet flat on the floor. Place your hands at the sides of your head to support your neck (or continue to use a towel if you prefer). Now pull your tummy in towards your spine and hold it in as you lift just the head and shoulders off the floor, then lower them again. Breathe out as you lift, and breathe in as you lower. Repeat 6 times slowly, then rest and repeat.

19 Back Strengthener Lie on your front, with both arms down at your sides. Keep looking at the floor and keep both feet firmly on the floor, as you gently lift your upper body off the floor. If you find this too difficult, go back to having your elbows close to your waist and the palms up in front. Do 4 repetitions, then rest and repeat.

22 Abdominal Stretch Lying on your front, place your bent arms in front of you and prop yourself up on your elbows, keeping the whole of each forearm on the floor. Now gently lift the chin forward slightly to feel a stretch down the front of the trunk. Hold for 6 seconds, then rest.

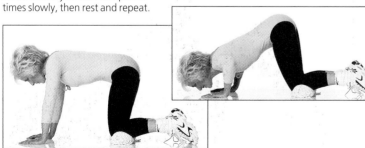

20 Press Ups Come up onto your hands and knees, still using a towel under the knees if you wish. Check that your hands are directly under your shoulders and that your knees are under your hips. Lower your forehead down in front of your hands, then come up again without locking out the elbows. Keep your tummy pulled in and your back flat. Do 8 repetitions, then rest and repeat.

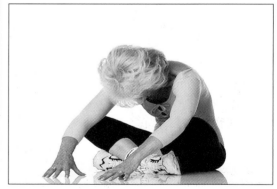

23 Spine Stretch Sit with your legs comfortably crossed and place your hands in front of you on the floor. Lower your head and slide the hands further along the floor to feel a stretch along your spine. Hold for 8 seconds, then release.

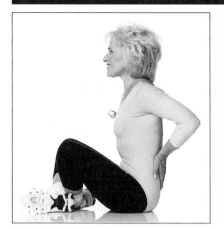

24 Chest Stretch Sit upright with legs still crossed. Place your hands in the small of your back and gently ease your shoulders back to feel a stretch across your chest. Hold for 8 seconds, then release.

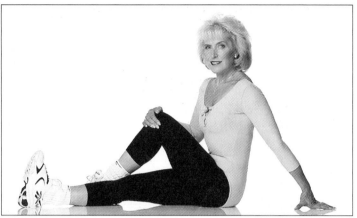

26 Outer Thigh Stretch Sit with both legs out in front, then cross your right leg over the left and place your right foot in line with the left knee. Now place your left hand on the outside of the right knee and the other hand on the floor for support. Gently squeeze the right knee further across the chest to feel a stretch in the outer thigh. Hold for 8 seconds, then release. Change legs and repeat.

POSITIVE THOUGHT FOR THE DAY

Reaching this third week is a very important and significant achievement. It is at this time that some do-gooders may make all kinds of suggestions. 'I heard you could eat any amount of steak and you'd lose loads of weight' or 'didn't I read somewhere that you aren't supposed to eat carbohydrate and protein at the same meal?' These views do not feature in my own dieting philosophy. What is absolutely vital is that while you are on one particular diet, you follow the rules that apply to that diet, and those rules only. The next time someone offers you advice on slimming – did they try it? Did it work for them? Are they slim now?

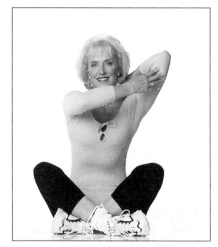

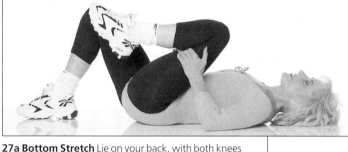

27a Bottom Stretch Lie on your back, with both knees bent and feet flat on the floor. Draw one knee into the chest, holding underneath the knee, and squeeze the raised leg towards the chest to feel a stretch in your bottom. Hold for 10 seconds, then move on to 27b.

27b Back of Thigh Stretch Now extend the leg further to feel the stretch move to the back of the thigh. Keep your hips on the floor and move one hand further up the leg for support. Hold for 10 seconds, then try to extend the knee a little further in order to develop the stretch more. Hold for a further 10 seconds, then release.

Repeat 27a and 27b on the other leg.

25 Tricep Stretch Sitting with legs crossed, head up and shoulders back, place your right hand behind your right shoulder and take the left hand across in front to push the arm further back. Hold for 6 seconds, then change sides and repeat.

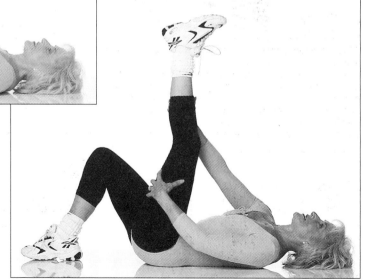

DAY 16

On previous days we have talked about setting goals. I firmly believe that we can accomplish so much more in our lives if we just pause occasionally to take stock of our plans and our aims. We all need a goal, and once we are well on the way to achieving it, then it is essential that we start thinking about another one. The greater the goal the better. It can be really ambitious but it must be realistic. Some goals will be short term (like your weight and inch loss campaign) and others will be longer term, such as changing your job or starting your own business. Start thinking today about what you would really like to work towards over the next few months and even years. If you want to achieve it badly enough, you can't fail to succeed!

—Menu—

BREAKFAST

25g (1oz) bran flakes mixed with 1 × 150g (5oz) diet yogurt and 1 chopped fresh pear (including the skin)

OR

2 bananas, sliced and topped with Total 0% Greek yogurt and 1 teaspoon strawberry preserve

LUNCH

4 slices of light bread spread with reduced-oil salad dressing and made into sandwiches with 75g (3oz) tinned salmon and sliced cucumber, plus a low-fat fromage frais

OR

200g (7oz) baked beans on 2 slices of wholemeal toast, plus 1 × 150g (5oz) diet yogurt .

DINNER

CHICKEN CHOP SUEY (see recipe, page 175)
PLUS
RASPBERRY AND STRAWBERRY BAVAROIS (see recipe, page 181)

OR

SPICED BEAN CASSEROLE (see recipe, page 183)
PLUS
CHOCOLATE AND COFFEE ROULADE (see recipe, page 175)

WARM UP – MOBILITY AND PULSE-RAISING

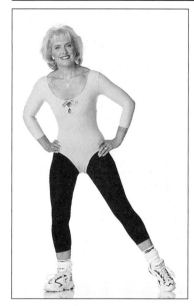

1 Weight Transfer Step out to the right, taking your weight on to the right foot and tapping the left toe to the floor with legs apart. Now transfer the weight to the left leg, tapping the right toe to the floor. Keep transferring your weight from one side to the other for 32 counts.

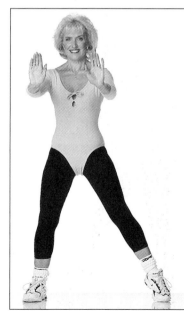

2 Double Steps with Arm Presses Take 2 steps to the right and, at the same time, press both arms out in front at chest height. Now take 2 steps back to the left. Keep your body upright, with your shoulders back and your head up. Repeat the sequence 4 times altogether.

3 Side Bends
Stand with feet apart and knees slightly bent. Now lean over to the right side, reaching out with the right arm and lifting the left elbow up. Come up to the centre and then lean to the other side. Keep the hips still throughout and try not to lean forward or back. Repeat 12 times altogether, changing sides each time.

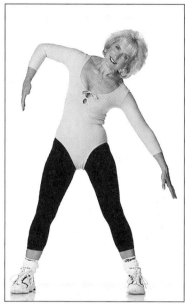

5 Ski Swings
Stand with feet together and lift your arms above your head. Pulling your tummy in tight and keeping your head up, swing down, bending your knees and taking the arms behind you as shown. Lift and lower under control 6 times altogether.

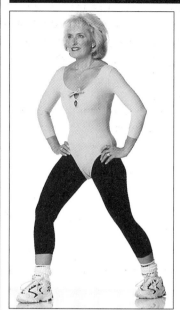

6 Calf Stretch Stand upright, with one foot in front of the other. Keep the back leg straight and bend the front leg and make sure both feet point forward. Lean towards the front leg to feel a stretch in the lower leg at the back. Now try to take the back leg further back to gain a more effective stretch. Hold for 8 seconds, then change legs and repeat.

4 Hip Rolls With feet wide apart and knees bent, roll the hips around in a full circle, from the side, round to the front, and then to the back. Keep it very smooth and under control. Repeat 4 times slowly in one direction, then change direction and repeat.

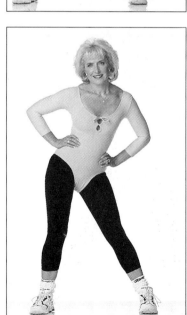

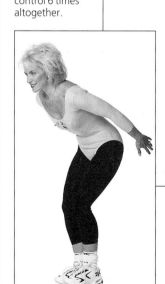

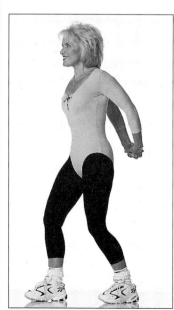

7 Lower Calf and Chest Stretch Place your right leg slightly behind the left leg and bend both knees. Keep both heels firmly on the floor and keep the hips tucked under to feel a stretch further down the calf on the right leg. Now take both hands and either clasp them behind you or place them in the small of your back and squeeze your shoulders back to feel a stretch across your chest. Keep your head up and your back straight at all times. Hold for 8 seconds, then release.

8 Lower Calf and Upper Back Stretch Place the left leg slightly behind the right leg and bend both knees. Keep both heels firmly on the floor and keep the hips tucked under to feel a stretch in the lower left leg. Now bring both arms round in front at chest height, drop your head forward and press your arms away from your upper back to feel a stretch in the upper back. Hold for 8 seconds, then release.

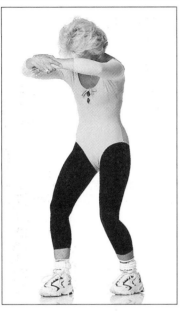

9 Back of Thigh Stretch Stand with your back leg bent and your front leg straight, and place your hands in the middle of your thighs. Now, keeping your head up and your back flat, lean forward until you feel a stretch in the back of the straight leg. Hold for 8 seconds, then change legs and repeat.

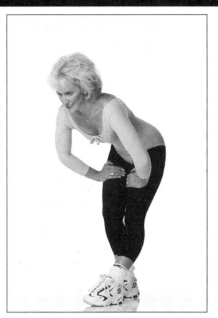

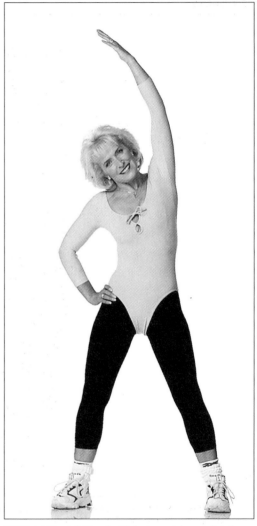

10 Front of Thigh Stretch Take hold around one ankle so that the knee points towards the floor and the knees are fairly close together. Try to keep the knee of the supporting leg slightly bent and push the hip forward on the held leg to feel the stretch down the front of the thigh. Hold for 8 seconds, then change legs and repeat.

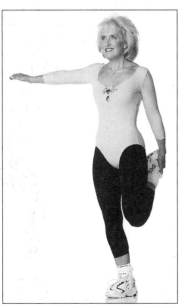

11 Inner Thigh Stretch Take the legs very wide and place one foot out diagonally, with the knee bent in line with the toes. The other leg is straight, with the foot pointing forward. To feel the stretch on the inside of the thigh, take the straight leg further away from you. Hold for 8 seconds, then change legs and repeat.

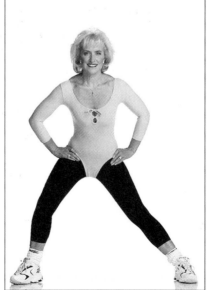

12 Waist Stretch Stand with feet apart, knees slightly bent and tummy pulled in. Now lift your right arm up above your head and place your left hand on the top of the left thigh. Bend slightly over to the left to feel a stretch down the waist on your right side. Try not to lean forward or back. Hold for 8 seconds, then release and repeat to the other side.

SEQUENCE 1

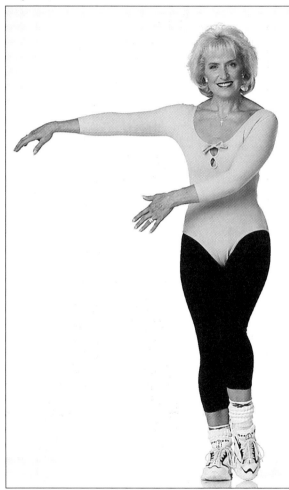

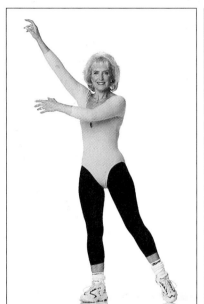

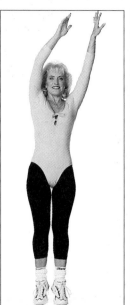

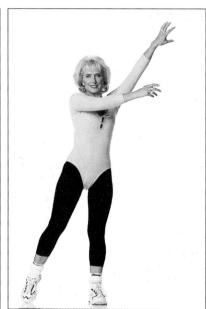

▲ **13b Travel Overs** Take the 2 steps to the side, swinging your arms over in the direction that you are moving. You should now be able to add a small jump as the feet come together in the middle, but make sure your heels land on the floor if you add this. Repeat twice to each side before moving on to 13c.

13a Step Touch Swing Step from side to side swinging the arms to just above shoulder height. Try to take wider steps now, with a deeper bend of the knees, but make sure you control the move and keep your head up and back straight. Repeat 8 times before moving on to 13b.

13c Touch Backs As you come back from the final travel over, take the right leg back to touch the floor with the toe, leaning forward slightly and pushing your arms out in front at the same time. Do 8 touch backs with alternate legs before moving on to Sequence 2.

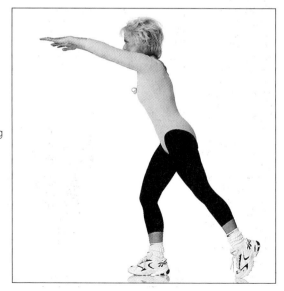

SEQUENCE 2

14a Hopscotch with Elbow Presses Take a step out to the side on the right leg and bend the left leg up behind. At the same time have your elbows up at shoulder height and, as the leg lifts at the back, press the elbows behind you, then repeat to the other side. Now make the steps wider and use the arms more strongly to make the move more effective. Do 8 times to alternate sides, then change to 14b.

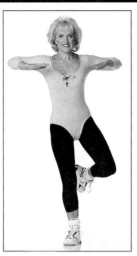

14b Walks with Rolling Arms Take 3 steps forward then clap, bringing the feet together on the 4th count, then take 3 steps back again. Roll the arms at chest height as you walk and now try to cover a lot more floor and keep tall. Repeat forward and back twice before moving on to 14c.

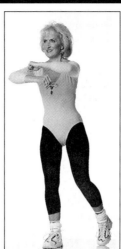

14c Skip Turns Take 4 counts to turn all the way round with a light skip, then go round the other way. Make sure the heels make contact with the floor and keep the trunk upright. Now move on to Sequence 3.

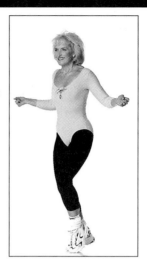

SEQUENCE 3

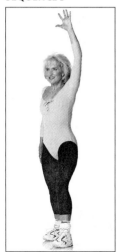

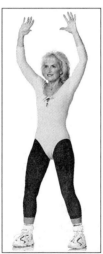

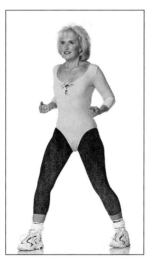

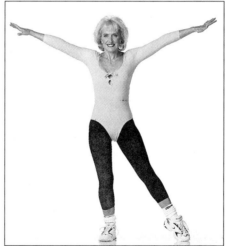

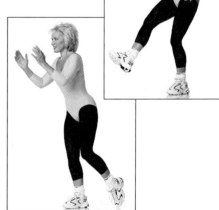

15a Box Step with High Arms Take a step forward with the right leg, leading with the heel, with the right arm overhead. Now do the same on the left side. As you step back with alternate legs, draw your elbows behind you at waist height with 2 little pushes. Step wide and use the arms strongly but keep your body upright. Do 4 box steps before moving on to 15b.

15b Half Jacks with Arms Take alternate toes out to the sides, bringing your arms out to just above shoulder height at the same time. As you change from one foot to the other add a small spring to increase the intensity of the move. Repeat 8 times under control before moving on to 15c.

15c Double Scoops with Claps On the last half jack, turn to your right and make a scooping action with both arms as you lead off with the heel of the right foot, bringing the left foot close up behind you. Take another scoop to the right, adding a clap at the end before turning to go left. Repeat a double scoop to each side again before starting again from Sequence 1.

Keep repeating the sequences from 1–3 until you feel you have done enough to challenge yourself.

16 Waist Curls Lie on your back with knees bent and feet flat on the floor. Place your right hand behind your head and extend your left arm out to the side on the floor at shoulder level. Pull your tummy in and hold it there as you lift your right shoulder across in the direction of the left leg. Only a small lift is necessary. Lower the shoulder again and repeat, breathing out as you lift and breathing in as you lower. Do 6 on this side, then change arms and repeat on the other side.

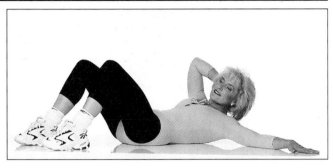

17 Inner Thigh Toner Lie on your side and place the top leg over the underneath leg, still using the towel under the knee for extra comfort. Smoothly lift the underneath leg, then lower it again. Repeat 12 times, then rest and repeat. Roll over and repeat with the other leg.

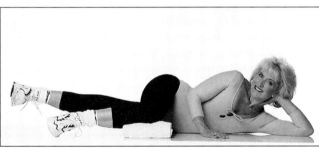

18 Upper Back Squeezes Lie on your front, with your arms by your sides. Keeping your head in contact with the floor, gently lift your shoulders up and back to feel the work across the shoulder blades, then release. Take your time to lift and lower so that you can keep the movement smooth. Repeat 6 times, then rest and repeat.

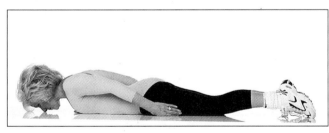

19 Outer Thigh Toner Lie on your side, propped on your elbow (or you can continue to use a towel if you prefer). The underneath leg is bent and the top leg is now straight, with the hips stacked on top of each other. Now lift the top leg to just above hip height, keeping the foot pointing forward and without tipping the hips back. Lower the leg again and repeat. Do 12 repetitions, then rest and repeat. Roll over and repeat with the other leg.

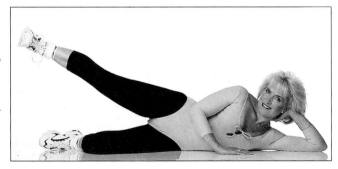

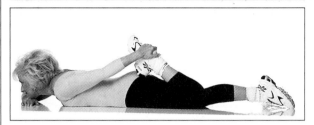

20 Front of Thigh Stretch Lie on your front, bend your right knee up and take hold of the ankle. Ease the heel close to the hip and push that hip firmly into the floor. Hold for 10 seconds, then change legs and repeat.

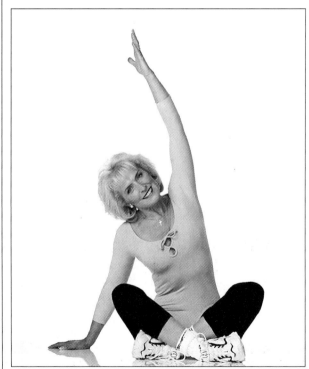

21 Waist Stretch Sit upright with legs comfortably crossed. Lift your right arm up in the air toward the ceiling and place your left hand on the floor for support. Now, keeping both hips firmly on the floor, lean slightly to the left to feel a stretch down the waist on the right side. Hold for 8 seconds, then release and repeat to the other side.

22 Upper Back Stretch Sitting cross-legged, bring both arms round in front of you at chest height and clasp your hands. Drop your head forward, and round your spine to feel a stretch across the back of the shoulders. Hold for 8 seconds, then release.

▼ **24 Outer Thigh Stretch** Sit with both legs out in front, then cross your right leg over the left and place your right foot in line with the left knee. Now place your left hand on the outside of the right knee and the other hand on the floor for support. Gently squeeze the right knee further across the chest to feel a stretch in the outer thigh. Hold for 8 seconds, then release. Change legs and repeat.

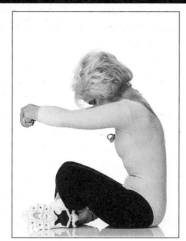

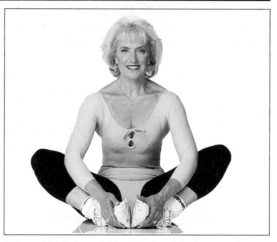

23 Inner Thigh Stretch Sit with soles of the feet together and your hands around your ankles. Now sit up tall and, with a straight back, lean forward slightly to place the elbows on the insides of the knees. Press down gently to feel a stretch on the insides of the thighs. Hold for 10 seconds, then try to press further to develop the stretch more. Hold for 10 more seconds, then release.

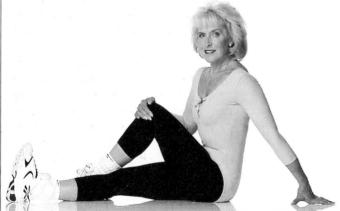

▶ **25 Back of Thigh Stretch** Lie on your back with knees bent and feet flat on the floor. Take hold behind one knee and extend the leg to feel the stretch in the back of the thigh. Keep your hips on the floor and move one hand further up the leg for support. Hold for 10 seconds, then try to extend the knee a little further in order to develop the stretch more. Hold for a further 10 seconds, then release and repeat with the other leg.

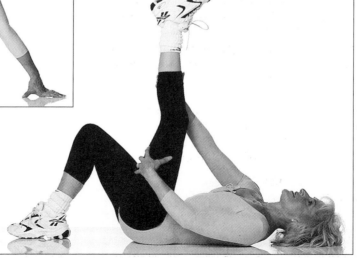

POSITIVE THOUGHT FOR THE DAY

This morning we talked about setting goals. I would like to suggest that you take a piece of paper and rule it as follows (see table on page 199) including the headings Short Term, Long Term and Ultimate Goals, and then separating them into two sections – Tangible and Intangible. Within each section add a couple of columns, heading the first one Target Date and the second one Date Achieved. Target Date can be a specific date or as general as just the month or year in which you hope to achieve that goal. You only fill in the Date Achieved after you have reached your goal weight. It doesn't matter if it is after the Target Date. The important factor is that you did it.

You don't have to show your master plan to anyone, but if you complete and update it periodically you will achieve so much more. If you want to do something badly enough and set about it seriously it is staggering how much help just seems to fall your way. So be bold in your plans, and even if you don't accomplish them all, those you do achieve are probably far more than you ever dreamed possible anyway.

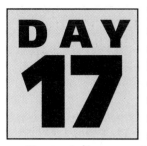

DAY 17

Did you give some serious thought to your goals? Don't worry if you couldn't think of many. It is fine to start off with just one or two very straightforward ones such as 'have my hair restyled' or 'buy a new dress' and perhaps 'take a holiday abroad next year'. As the days go by, open your mind to what is going on around you — what are other people's goals. It is always wise to look towards those who inspire and impress you. Are you happy in your job? Could it be better? How can you improve the way things are? Approach it one step at a time — in the same way you are reducing your weight and inches.

You are going to reach your weight and inch loss target, and when you do, unless you have another goal to aim for, you may well let your fitness campaign relax and fall back into your old habits. As you have another rest day from the exercises today, start thinking about new physical activities you could try.

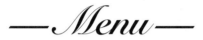
—Menu—

BREAKFAST

HOME-MADE MUESLI (see recipe, page 178)

OR

PINEAPPLE BOAT (see recipe, page 180)

LUNCH

Stir 1 teaspoon of curry powder into 75g (3oz) plain yogurt and mix with 115g (4oz) chopped chicken or turkey breast. Serve with salad and 75g (3oz) cooked weight cold boiled brown rice, plus 1 orange

OR

Jacket potato (approx.175g/6oz) topped with chopped peppers and onion mixed with 50g (2oz) low-fat cottage cheese, plus 1 × 150g (5oz) diet yogurt

DINNER

1 trout stuffed with 75g (3oz) prawns and steamed, microwaved or grilled. Serve with unlimited potatoes and other vegetables

PLUS

50g (2oz) Wall's 'Too Good To Be True' frozen dessert

OR

STUFFED PEPPERS (see recipe, page 183)

PLUS

RASPBERRY MOUSSE (see recipe, page 181)

POSITIVE THOUGHT FOR THE DAY

I hope your mind has been working in an expansive way and that you have thought more about your future.

Before I became involved in business, I really had very few goals, with the result that I didn't get very far. Then suddenly I got a bit more confidence, I felt better about my weight, my husband encouraged me as I started out in various career directions, and goals actually began to emerge. It is quite incredible what has happened in my life – the help that has just seemed to come, the opportunities that have arisen, the doors that have opened in all directions – and if occasionally one closed, it didn't matter because it always meant a better one would open later.

So don't ever dismiss anything as impossible. Even if you try at something and fail the first time, have another go. You will have a much better chance of success next time because you will have learnt from your previous experience. If you have a positive attitude to life you will get there in the end.

DAY 18

Are you feeling slimmer each day or do you feel things have slowed up? Inevitably, once we have established ourselves into a new way of eating, progress does seem a little slower. I do hope you took a photograph of yourself before you started. If you look back at it you will see what a transformation has already taken place. And whenever you wonder whether this regime is still working, just consult your Weight and Inch Loss Record Chart and try on your measuring garment.

It is very strange that the slimmer we get, the more critical we become of our bodies, often exclaiming 'but I've still got a big waist/tummy/hips/bottom'. Even those people who slim right down to their goal weight will always find parts they wish were even slimmer! We have to be realistic, but we should always remember the progress we've made.

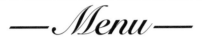
—Menu—

BREAKFAST

3 slices of light bread topped with 200g (7oz) baked beans

OR

225g (8oz) seedless grapes served on ½ a honeydew melon, plus 1 × 150g (5oz) diet yogurt

LUNCH

450g (1lb) any fresh fruit of your choice, plus 1 × 150g (5oz) diet yogurt

OR

115g (4oz) red kidney beans, 115g (4oz) sweetcorn and unlimited chopped cucumber, tomatoes and spring onions all tossed in mint sauce then mixed with plain yogurt and served on a bed of lettuce, plus ½ a fresh grapefruit

DINNER

115g (4oz) gammon steak (all fat removed) served with a slice of pineapple, 115g (4oz) potatoes and unlimited other vegetables
PLUS
AUTUMN PUDDING (see recipe, page 173)

OR

CHICKPEA AND FENNEL CASSEROLE (see recipe, page 175)
PLUS
1 banana sliced lengthways, filled with 115g (4oz) fresh or frozen raspberries or blackcurrants and topped with 50g (2oz) diet yogurt

WARM UP – MOBILITY AND PULSE-RAISING

1 Grapevine You will be doing this new move in the aerobics session, so you need to practise it slowly here in the warm up. If you find it difficult, then simply take 2 steps to the side instead.

Take a step to the right with the right leg (1a) and cross the left leg behind it (1b). Now continue moving to the right with another step (1c) and finally bring the left foot to the right foot to finish the move (1d). Start slow, but then try to perform it more quickly and rhythmically. Repeat 8 times.

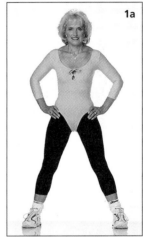
1a

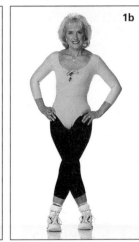
1b

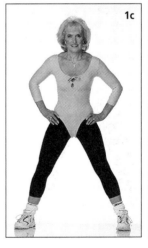
1c

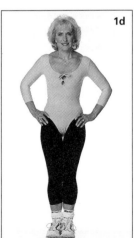
1d

2 Weight Transfer with Arm Circles
Transfer your weight from one foot to the other and at the same time take the opposite arm in a circling action just above the head. So, as you take the weight to the right leg, the left arm goes over and so on. Control the move and pull your tummy in and maintain a good posture. Repeat 16 times altogether.

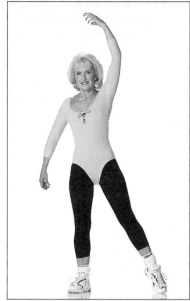

3 Ski Swings Stand with feet together and lift your arms above your head. Pulling your tummy in tight and keeping your head up, swing down, bending your knees and taking the arms behind you as shown. Lift and lower under control 6 times altogether.

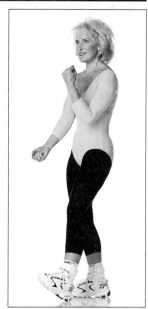

5 Heel/Toe with Bicep Curls Take the right heel out diagonally in front on the floor and then change to the toe. At the same time bend alternate elbows, keeping them close to the waist and under control. Rhythmically keep changing from heel to toe for 4 counts, counting 1 every time the heel strikes the floor. Change legs and repeat, then repeat again on each leg.

4 Waist Twists Stand with feet apart, tummy pulled in tight and knees slightly bent. Bring your arms up to shoulder height as shown then twist to alternate sides from the waist, keeping your hips still. Do 8 repetitions slowly and under control.

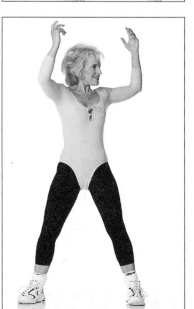

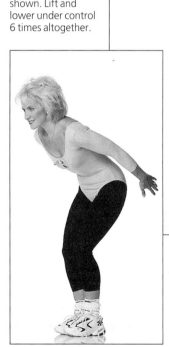

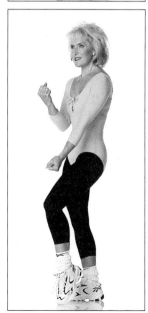

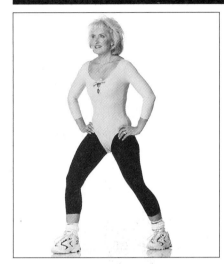

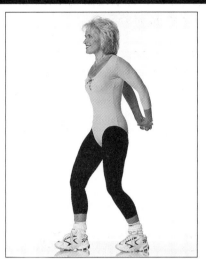

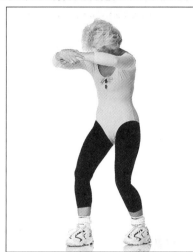

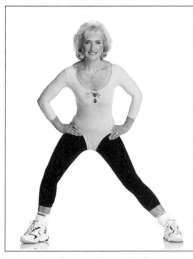

6 Calf Stretch Stand upright, with one foot in front of the other. Keep the back leg straight and bend the front leg and make sure both feet point forward. Lean towards the front leg to feel a stretch in the lower leg at the back. Now try to take the back leg further back to gain a more effective stretch. Hold for 8 seconds, then change legs and repeat.

7 Lower Calf and Chest Stretch Place your right leg slightly behind the left leg and bend both knees. Keep both heels firmly on the floor and keep the hips tucked under to feel a stretch further down the calf on the right leg. Now take both hands and either clasp them behind you or place them in the small of your back and squeeze your shoulders back to feel a stretch across your chest. Keep your head up and your back straight at all times. Hold for 8 seconds, then release.

8 Lower Calf and Upper Back Stretch Place the left leg slightly behind the right leg and bend both knees. Keep both heels firmly on the floor and keep the hips tucked under to feel a stretch in the lower left leg. Now bring both arms round in front at chest height, drop your head forward and press your arms away from your upper back to feel a stretch in the upper back. Hold for 8 seconds, then release.

9 Inner Thigh Stretch Take the legs very wide and place one foot out diagonally, with the knee bent in line with the toes. The other leg is straight, with the foot pointing forward. To feel the stretch on the inside of the thigh, take the straight leg further away from you. Hold for 8 seconds, then change legs and repeat.

10 Tricep Stretch Standing with feet apart, tummy pulled in tight and knees slightly bent, take your right hand behind the right shoulder and use the left hand on the fleshy part of the right underarm to push it further back. Keep your head up throughout and hold for 8 seconds. Change arms and repeat.

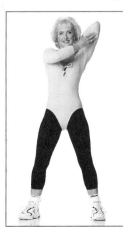

11 Back of Thigh Stretch Stand with your back leg bent and your front leg straight, and place your hands in the middle of your thighs. Now, keeping your head up and your back flat, lean forward until you feel a stretch in the back of the straight leg. Hold for 8 seconds, then change legs and repeat.

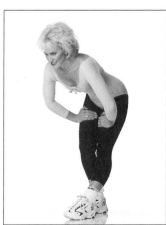

12 Front of Thigh Stretch Take hold around one ankle so that the knee points toward the floor and the knees are fairly close together. Try to keep the knee of the supporting leg slightly bent and push the hip forward on the held leg to feel the stretch down the front of the thigh. Hold for 8 seconds, then change legs and repeat.

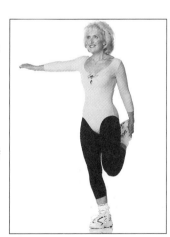

Another sequence is added now, as you should be very familiar with all the moves and ready for something different.

SEQUENCE 1

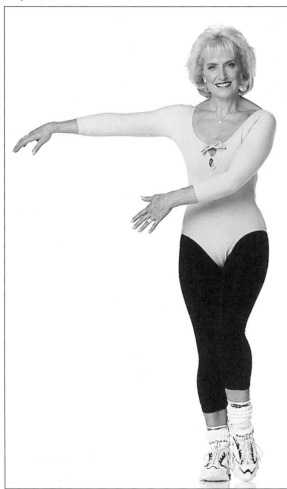

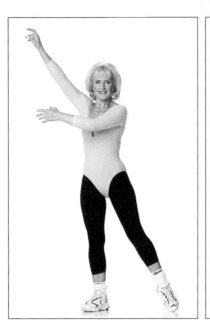

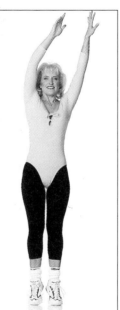

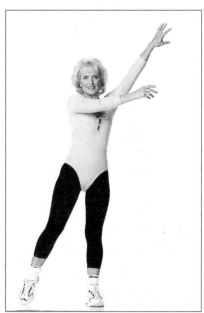

▲**13b Travel Overs** Take the 2 steps to the side, swinging your arms over in the direction that you are moving. You should now be able to add a small jump as the feet come together in the middle, but make sure your heels land on the floor if you add this. Repeat twice to each side before moving on to 13c.

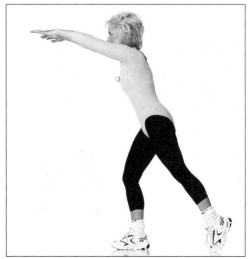

13c Touch Backs As you come back from the final travel over, take the right leg back to touch the floor with the toe, leaning forward slightly and pushing your arms out in front at the same time. Do 8 touch backs with alternate legs before moving on to Sequence 2.

13a Step Touch Swing Step from side to side swinging the arms to just above shoulder height. Try to take wider steps now, with a deeper bend of the knees, but make sure you control the move and keep your head up and back straight. Repeat 8 times before moving on to 13b.

SEQUENCE 2

14a Hopscotch with Elbow Presses Take a step out to the side on the right leg and bend the left leg up behind. At the same time have your elbows up at shoulder height and, as the leg lifts at the back, press the elbows behind you, then repeat to the other side. Now make the steps wider and use the arms more strongly to make the move more effective. Do 8 times to alternate sides, then change to 14b.

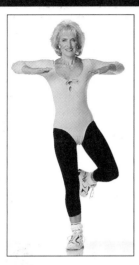

14b Walks with Rolling Arms Take 3 steps forward then clap, bringing the feet together on the 4th count, then take 3 steps back again. Roll the arms at chest height as you walk and now try to cover a lot more floor and keep tall. Repeat forward and back twice before moving on to 14c.

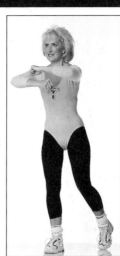

4c Skip Turns Take 4 counts to turn all the way round with a light skip, then go round the other way. Make sure the heels make contact with the floor and keep the trunk upright. Now move on to Sequence 3.

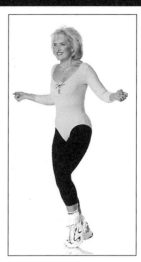

SEQUENCE 3

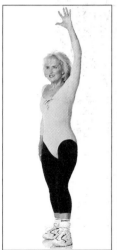
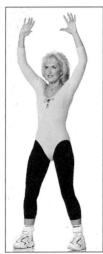
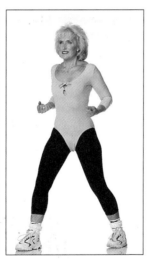

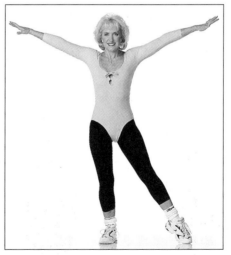

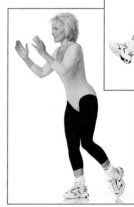

15a Box Step with High Arms Take a step forward with the right leg, leading with the heel, with the right arm overhead. As you step back with alternate legs, draw your elbows behind you at waist height with 2 little pushes. Step wide and use the arms strongly but keep your body upright. Do 4 box steps before moving on to 15b.

15b Half Jacks with Arms Take alternate toes out to the sides, bringing your arms out to just above shoulder height at the same time. As you change from one foot to the other add a small spring to increase the intensity of the move. Repeat 8 times under control before moving on to 15c.

15c Double Scoops with Claps On the last half jack, turn to your right and make a scooping action with both arms as you lead off with the heel of the right foot, bringing the left foot close up behind you. Take another scoop to the right, adding a clap at the end before turning to go left. Repeat a double scoop to each side again before moving on to Sequence 4.

SEQUENCE 4

16a Grapevine with Arm Circles Take a grapevine to your right and as the feet come together at the end take 2 knee bends with a little jump off the floor, circling the arms in front of you at the same time. Now take a grapevine back to the left with 2 knee bends and arm circles on the end. Repeat twice through before moving on to 16b.

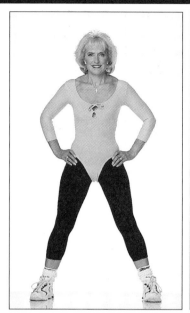

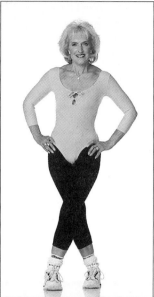

16b Alternate Squats with Jumps Next take a large squat step out to the right, really bending your knees and taking your hips back. As you come up again bring the feet together and do 2 small jumps with claps. Now do exactly the same out to the left. Keep your head up and your back straight all the time. Repeat 4 times altogether.

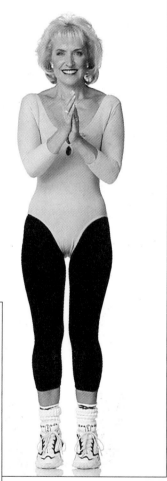

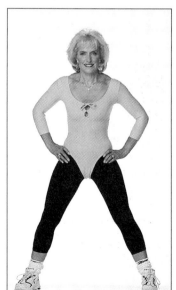

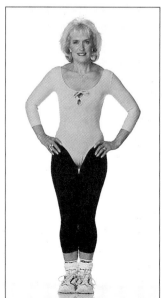

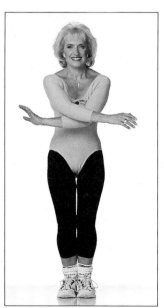

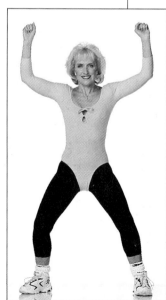

Keep repeating the sequences from 1–4 until you feel you have done enough to challenge yourself.

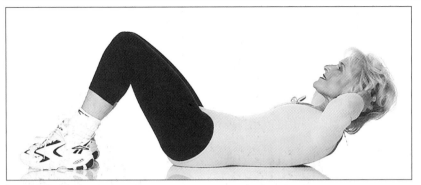

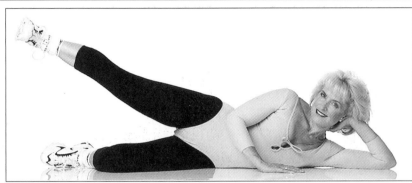

17 Abdominal Curl Lie on your back, with your knees bent and your feet flat on the floor. Place your hands at the sides of your head to support your neck (or continue to use a towel if you prefer). Now pull your tummy in towards your spine and hold it in as you lift just the head and shoulders off the floor, then lower them again. Breathe out as you lift, and breathe in as you lower. Repeat 6 times slowly, then rest and repeat.

18 Outer Thigh Toner Lie on your side, propped on your elbow (or you can continue to use a towel if you prefer). The underneath leg is bent and the top leg is now straight, with the hips stacked on top of each other. Now lift the top leg to just above hip height, keeping the foot pointing forward and without tipping the hips back. Lower the leg again and repeat. Do 12 repetitions, then rest and repeat. Roll over and repeat with the other leg.

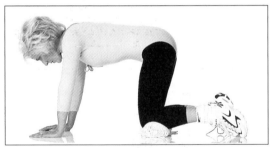

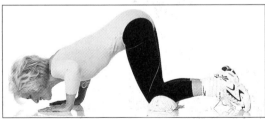

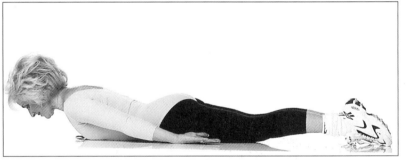

20 Back Strengthener Lie on your front, with both arms down at your sides. Keep looking at the floor and keep both feet firmly on the floor, as you gently lift your upper body off the floor. If you find this too difficult, go back to having your elbows close to your waist and the palms up in front. Do 4 repetitions, then rest and repeat.

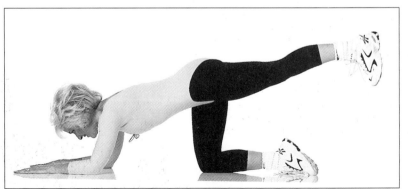

21 Bottom Toner Come up onto your forearms and knees, and place a towel under the knees if it helps. Pull your tummy in tightly and extend one leg out behind you with the toe on the floor. Now lift the leg under control to just above hip height and then lower it again. Keep both hips facing the floor and take care not to swing the leg. Do 12 repetitions, then change legs and repeat.

19 Press Ups Come up onto your hands and knees, still using a towel under the knees if you wish. Check that your hands are directly under your shoulders and that your knees are under your hips. Lower your forehead down in front of your hands, then come up again without locking out the elbows. Keep your tummy pulled in and your back flat. Do 8 repetitions, then rest and repeat.

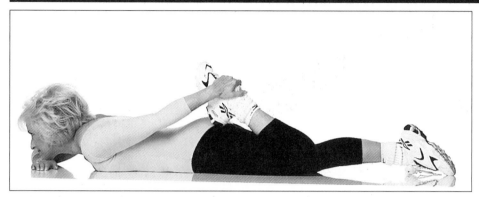

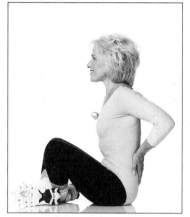

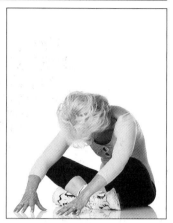

22 Front of Thigh Stretch Lie on your front, bend your right knee up and take hold of the ankle. Ease the heel close to the hip and push that hip firmly into the floor. Hold for 10 seconds, then change legs and repeat.

24 Chest Stretch Sit upright with legs still crossed. Place your hands in the small of your back and gently ease your shoulders back to feel a stretch across your chest. Hold for 8 seconds, then release.

25 Spine Stretch Sitting with legs comfortably crossed, place your hands in front of you on the floor. Lower your head and slide the hands further along the floor to feel a stretch along your spine. Hold for 8 seconds, then release.

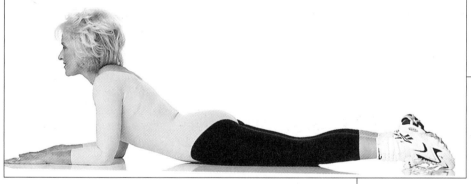

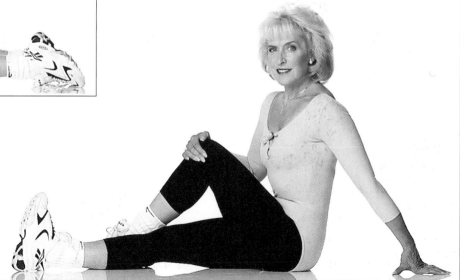

23 Abdominal Stretch Lying on your front, place your bent arms in front of you and prop yourself up on your elbows, keeping the whole of each forearm on the floor. Now gently lift the chin forward slightly to feel a stretch down the front of the trunk. Hold for 6 seconds, then rest.

26 Outer Thigh Stretch Sit with both legs out in front, then cross your right leg over the left and place your right foot in line with the left knee. Now place your left hand on the outside of the right knee and the other hand on the floor for support. Gently squeeze the right knee further across the chest to feel a stretch in the outer thigh. Hold for 8 seconds, then release. Change legs and repeat.

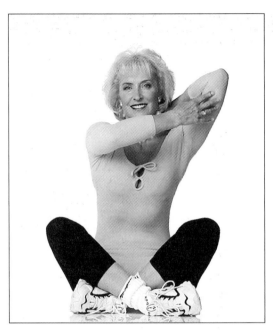

27 Tricep Stretch Sit with legs crossed, head up and shoulders back. Place your right hand behind your right shoulder and take the left hand across in front to push the arm further back. Hold for 6 seconds, then change sides and repeat.

28a Bottom Stretch Lie on your back, with both knees bent and feet flat on the floor. Draw one knee into the chest, holding underneath the knee, and squeeze the raised leg towards the chest to feel a stretch in your bottom. Hold for 10 seconds, then move on to 28b.

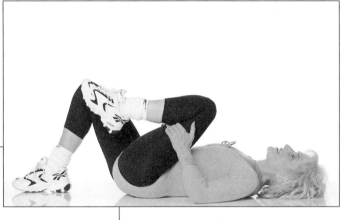

28b Back of Thigh Stretch Now extend the leg further to feel the stretch move to the back of the thigh. Keep your hips on the floor and move one hand further up the leg for support. Hold for 10 seconds, then try to extend the knee a little further in order to develop the stretch more. Hold for a further 10 seconds, then release.

Repeat 28a and 28b on the other leg.

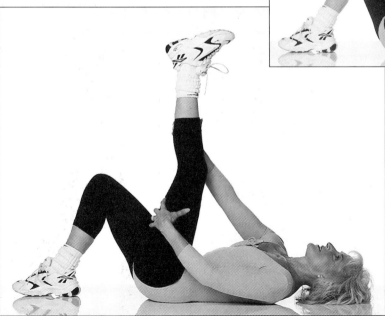

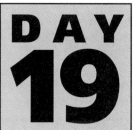

DAY 19

Only 2 days to go before you complete your third week of this New Inch Loss Plan. Do you feel really determined to reach the end of this programme? If you do, it will be the first fulfilment of a real goal – the first one of many! Not only will you feel a sense of achievement but you will also have re-educated your way of eating and the way you think about yourself. And you will look so much better – slimmer, fitter, healthier, with more confidence and vitality – all wonderful improvements in your life.

But life (and particularly slimming) is never plain sailing. There will be times when our good intentions fail miserably and we feel very disillusioned. This is normal! If we succeeded first time in everything we attempted, what challenges would be left? Even if you do cheat and eat something you shouldn't, it doesn't mean that you have failed on the New Inch Loss Plan. Far from it. All it means is that you will take slightly longer to achieve your goal – that's all.

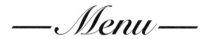

—Menu—

BREAKFAST

$^{1}/_{2}$ a fresh grapefruit, plus 50g (2oz) lean ham (all fat removed) served with a little mustard, 2 fresh tomatoes and 25g (1oz) bread

OR

5 prunes in natural juice served with 15g ($^{1}/_{2}$oz) bran flakes and 50g (2oz) low-fat fromage frais

LUNCH

4 brown Ryvitas spread with Branston pickle, topped with 50g (2oz) wafer thin chicken or turkey and served with salad, plus 115g (4oz) any fresh fruit

OR

4 × 150g (4 × 5oz) diet yogurts, plus 1 piece of any fresh fruit

DINNER

FISH PIE (see recipe, page 177)
PLUS
115g (4oz) peaches or any tinned fruit (in natural juice) and 1 × 150g (5oz) diet yogurt

OR

STUFFED MARROW (see recipe, page 183)
PLUS
225g (8oz) stewed fruit (no sugar) topped with a low-fat fromage frais

WARM UP – MOBILITY AND PULSE-RAISING

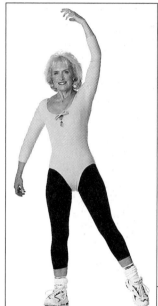

1 Weight Transfer with Arm Circles Transfer your weight from one foot to the other and at the same time take the opposite arm in a circling action just above the head. So, as you take the weight to the right leg, the left arm goes over and so on. Control the move and pull your tummy in and maintain a good posture. Repeat 16 times altogether.

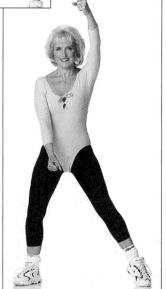

2 Side Steps with Monkey Arms Take 2 steps out to the right, with your arms straight out in front, pulling them up and down alternately in rhythm with the steps. Take 2 steps back to the left and keep going, to repeat the sequence 4 times altogether.

3 Side Bends Stand with feet apart and knees slightly bent. Now lean over to the right side, reaching out with the right arm and lifting the left elbow up. Come up to the centre and then lean to the other side. Keep the hips still throughout and try not to lean forward or back. Repeat 12 times altogether, changing sides each time.

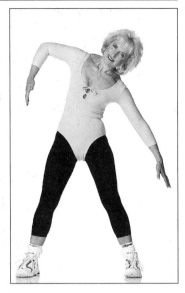

▼ **4 Half Jacks with Arms** Stand with a good posture and take the right foot out to the side, touching the floor with just the toe. At the same time lift both arms to just above shoulder height. Bring the feet together and repeat to the other side. Repeat 16 times.

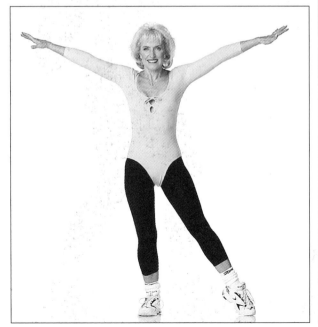

5 Waist Stretch Stand with feet apart, knees slightly bent and tummy pulled in. Now lift your right arm up above your head and place your left hand on the top of the left thigh. Bend slightly over to the left to feel a stretch down the waist on your right side. Try not to lean forward or back. Hold for 8 seconds, then release and repeat to the other side.

▼ **6 Inner Thigh Stretch** Take the legs very wide and place one foot out diagonally, with the knee bent in line with the toes. The other leg is straight, with the foot pointing forward. To feel the stretch on the inside of the thigh, take the straight leg further away from you. Hold for 8 seconds, then change legs and repeat.

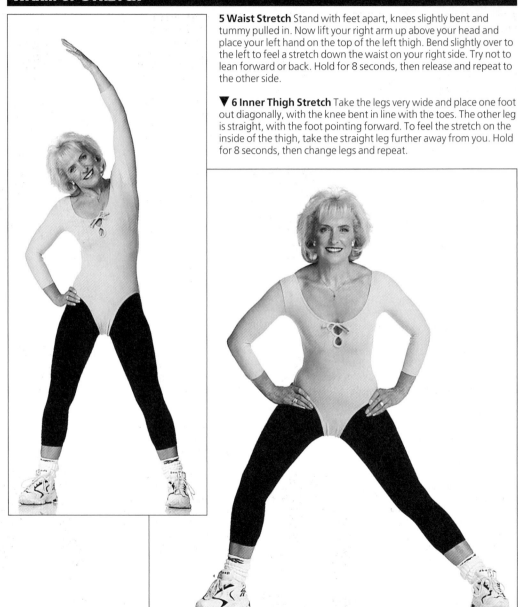

7 Front of Thigh Stretch Stand up straight and take hold around one ankle so that the knee points towards the floor and the knees are fairly close together. Try to keep the knee of the supporting leg slightly bent and push the hip forward on the held leg to feel the stretch down the front of the thigh. Hold for 8 seconds, then change legs and repeat.

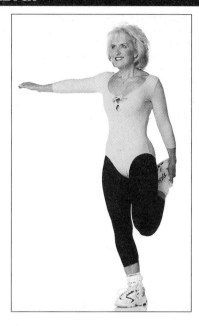

8 Calf Stretch Stand upright, with one foot in front of the other. Keep the back leg straight and bend the front leg and make sure both feet point forward. Lean towards the front leg to feel a stretch in the lower leg at the back. Now try to take the back leg further back to gain a more effective stretch. Hold for 8 seconds, then change legs and repeat.

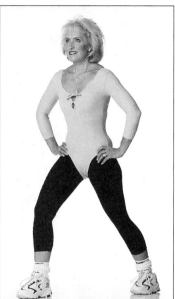

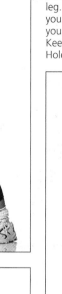

▼ **9 Lower Calf and Chest Stretch** Place your right leg slightly behind the left leg and bend both knees. Keep both heels firmly on the floor and keep the hips tucked under to feel a stretch further down the calf on the right leg. Now take both hands and either clasp them behind you or place them in the small of your back and squeeze your shoulders back to feel a stretch across your chest. Keep your head up and your back straight at all times. Hold for 8 seconds, then release.

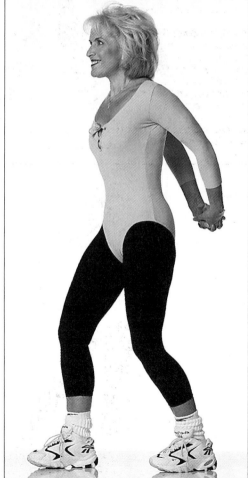

10 Lower Calf and Upper Back Stretch Place the left leg slightly behind the right leg and bend both knees. Keep both heels firmly on the floor and keep the hips tucked under to feel a stretch in the lower left leg. Now bring both arms round in front at chest height, drop your head forward and press your arms away from your upper back to feel a stretch in the upper back. Hold for 8 seconds, then release.

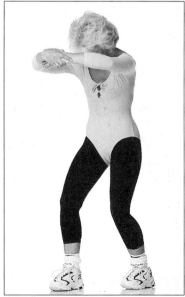

11 Tricep Stretch Stand with feet apart, tummy pulled in tight and knees slightly bent. Now take your right hand behind the right shoulder and use the left hand on the fleshy part of the right underarm to push it further back. Keep your head up throughout and hold for 6 seconds. Change arms and repeat.

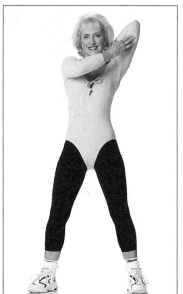

SEQUENCE 1

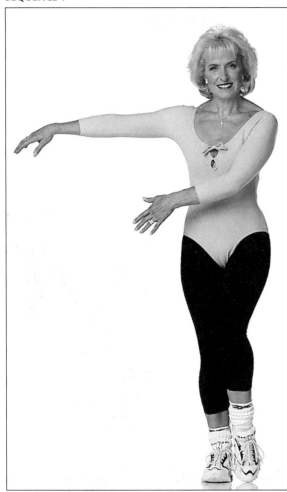

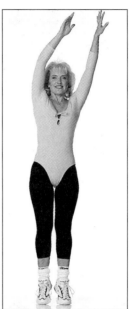

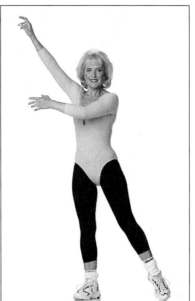

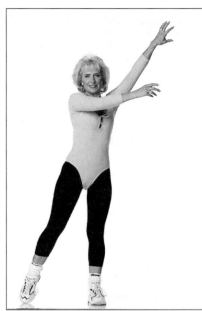

▲ **12b Travel Overs** Take the 2 steps to the side, swinging your arms over in the direction that you are moving. You should now be able to add a small jump as the feet come together in the middle, but make sure your heels land on the floor if you add this. Repeat twice to each side before moving on to 12c.

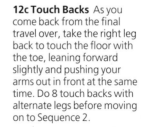

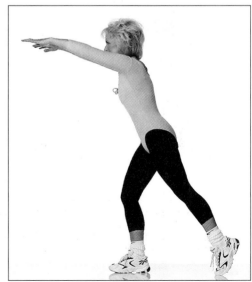

12c Touch Backs As you come back from the final travel over, take the right leg back to touch the floor with the toe, leaning forward slightly and pushing your arms out in front at the same time. Do 8 touch backs with alternate legs before moving on to Sequence 2.

12a Step Touch Swing Step from side to side swinging the arms to just above shoulder height. Try to take wider steps now, with a deeper bend of the knees, but make sure you control the move and keep your head up and back straight. Repeat 8 times before moving on to 12b.

SEQUENCE 2

13a Hopscotch with Elbow Presses Take a step out to the side on the right leg and bend the left leg up behind. At the same time have your elbows up at shoulder height and, as the leg lifts at the back, press the elbows behind you, then repeat to the other side. Now make the steps wider and use the arms more strongly to make the move more effective. Do 8 times to alternate sides, then change to 13b.

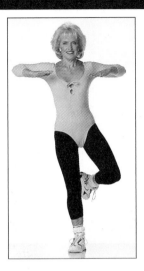

13b Walks with Rolling Arms Take 3 steps forward then clap, bringing the feet together on the 4th count, then take 3 steps back again. Roll the arms at chest height as you walk and now try to cover a lot more floor and keep tall. Repeat forward and back twice before moving on to 13c.

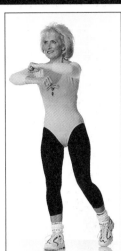

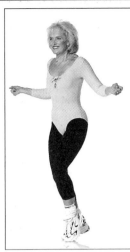

13c Skip Turns Take 4 counts to turn all the way round with a light skip, then go round the other way. Make sure the heels make contact with the floor and keep the trunk upright. Now move on to Sequence 3.

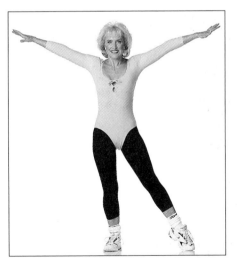

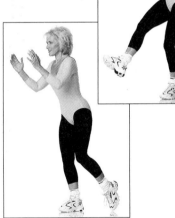

SEQUENCE 3

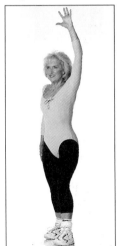

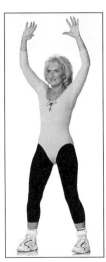

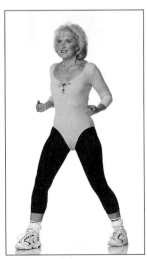

14a Box Step with High Arms Take a step forward with the right leg, leading with the heel, with the right arm overhead. As you step back with alternate legs, draw your elbows behind you at waist height with 2 little pushes. Step wide and use the arms strongly but keep your body upright. Do 4 box steps before moving on to 14b.

14b Half Jacks with Arms Take alternate toes out to the sides, bringing your arms out to just above shoulder height at the same time. As you change from one foot to the other add a small spring to increase the intensity of the move. Repeat 8 times under control before moving on to 14c.

14c Double Scoops with Claps On the last half jack, turn to your right and make a scooping action with both arms as you lead off with the heel of the right foot, bringing the left foot close up behind you. Take another scoop to the right, adding a clap at the end before turning to go left. Repeat a double scoop to each side again before moving on to Sequence 4.

SEQUENCE 4

15a Grapevine with Arm Circles Take a grapevine to your right and as the feet come together at the end take 2 knee bends with a little jump off the floor, circling the arms in front of you at the same time. Now take a grapevine back to the left with 2 knee bends and arm circles on the end. Repeat twice through before moving on to 15b.

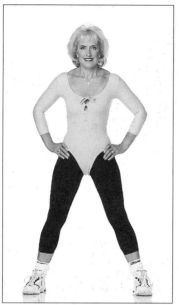
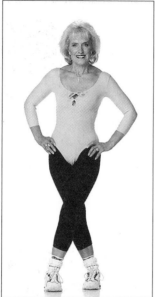

15b Alternate Squats with Jumps Next take a large squat step out to the right, really bending your knees and taking your hips back. As you come up again bring the feet together and do 2 small jumps with claps. Now do exactly the same out to the left. Keep your head up and your back straight all the time. Repeat 4 times altogether before starting again from Sequence 1.

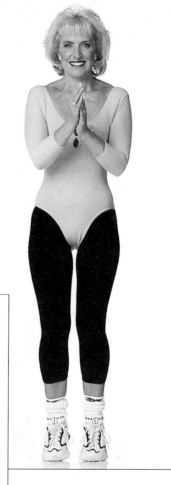

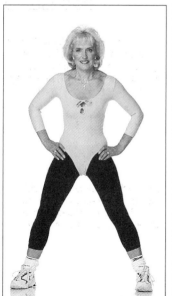
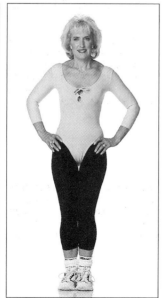
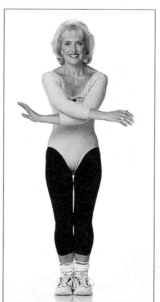
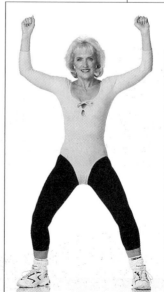

Keep repeating the sequences from 1–4 until you feel you have done enough to challenge yourself.

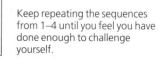

16 Waist Curls Lie on your back with knees bent and feet flat on the floor. Place your right hand behind your head and extend your left arm out to the side on the floor at shoulder level. Pull your tummy in and hold it there as you lift your right shoulder across in the direction of the left leg. Only a small lift is necessary. Lower the shoulder again and repeat, breathing out as you lift and breathing in as you lower. Do 6 on this side, then change arms and repeat on the other side.

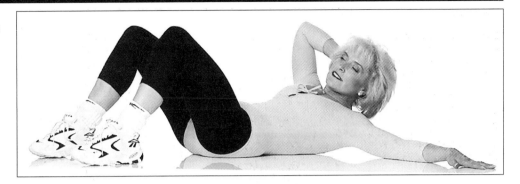

▶ **17 Inner Thigh Toner** Lie on your side and place the top leg over the underneath leg, still using the towel under the knee for extra comfort. Smoothly lift the underneath leg, then lower it again. Repeat 12 times, then rest and repeat. Roll over and repeat with the other leg.

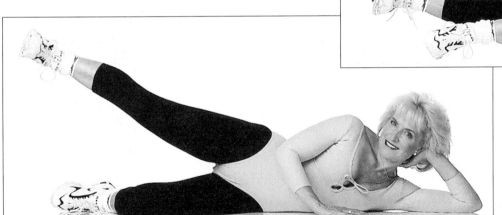

◀ **18 Outer Thigh Toner** Lie on your side, propped on your elbow. The underneath leg is bent and the top leg is now straight, with the hips stacked on top of each other. Now lift the top leg to just above hip height, keeping the foot pointing forward and without tipping the hips back. Lower the leg again and repeat. Do 12 repetitions, then rest and repeat. Roll over and repeat with the other leg.

19 Upper Back Squeezes Lie on your front, with your arms by your sides. Keeping your head in contact with the floor, gently lift your shoulders up and back to feel the work across the shoulder blades, then release. Take your time to lift and lower so that you can keep the movement smooth. Repeat 6 times, then rest and repeat.

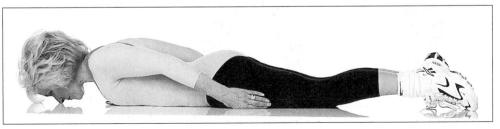

20 Front of Thigh Stretch Lie on your front, bend your right knee up and take hold of the ankle. Ease the heel close to the hip and push that hip firmly into the floor. Hold for 10 seconds, then change legs and repeat.

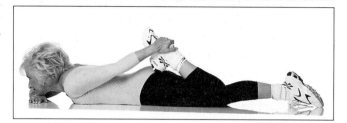

21 Waist Stretch Sit upright with legs comfortably crossed. Lift your right arm up in the air toward the ceiling and place your left hand on the floor for support. Now, keeping both hips firmly on the floor, lean slightly to the left to feel a stretch down the waist on the right side. Hold for 8 seconds, then release and repeat to the other side.

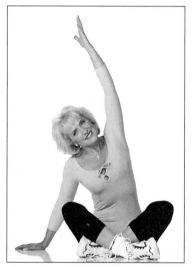

22 Upper Back Stretch Sitting cross-legged, bring both arms round in front of you at chest height and clasp your hands. Drop your head forward, and round your spine to feel a stretch across the back of the shoulders. Hold for 8 seconds, then release.

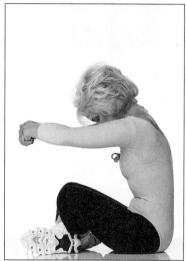

23 Inner Thigh Stretch Sit with soles of the feet together and your hands around your ankles. Now sit up tall and, with a straight back, lean forward slightly to place the elbows on the insides of the knees. Press down gently to feel a stretch on the insides of the thighs. Hold for 10 seconds, then try to press further to develop the stretch more. Hold for 10 more seconds, then release.

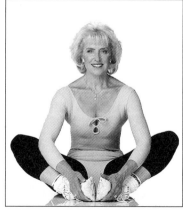

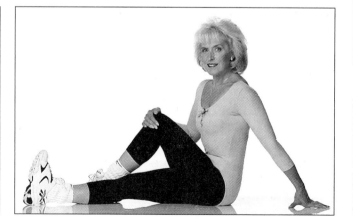

POSITIVE THOUGHT FOR THE DAY

I am certain that by now you will be able to see a significant improvement in your body. Look for the muscle tone and feel the muscles as you perform the exercises. On the first day, I doubt whether you could feel them at all!

Carrying on from this morning's thoughts about making the occasional slip while following the programme, we should also realise that this will happen as we attempt to achieve our other goals in life. We will find ourselves missing golden opportunities, getting ourselves involved in time-consuming, time-wasting activities which distract us from our main goals. Don't worry about this but learn from it. So long as we learn something from every mistake we make, the time hasn't been wasted.

24 Outer Thigh Stretch Sit with both legs out in front, then cross your right leg over the left and place your right foot in line with the left knee. Now place your left hand on the outside of the right knee and the other hand on the floor for support. Gently squeeze the right knee further across the chest to feel a stretch in the outer thigh. Hold for 8 seconds, then release. Change legs and repeat.

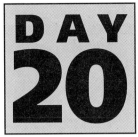

DAY 20

Yesterday we talked about the odd lapse in our good intentions to be a saintly slimmer, and also that occasionally our best intentions to achieve a goal are stifled – sometimes through our own wrong judgement but more often by getting involved in time-wasting, non-productive activities. Beware of finding yourself volunteering for all kinds of jobs that you don't want to do.

I am not suggesting that sometimes it is not totally appropriate to go and help someone. Children particularly appreciate a parent's involvement in a variety of projects. Husbands and wives also appreciate their partner's assistance. Hopefully, those closest to us have goals as well and I am sure we are all anxious to help them achieve them, just as we hope they want us to achieve ours.

Today you can take another rest day from the formal exercise programme, but stay active. Remember, it's weighing and measuring day the day after tomorrow, so please be super-good today!

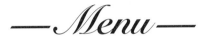

—Menu—

BREAKFAST

1 whole grapefruit, plus 150g (5oz) diet yogurt and 1 banana

OR

115g (4oz) baked beans and 115g (4oz) tinned tomatoes on 1 slice of wholemeal toast

LUNCH

1 slimmer's cup-a-soup and 1 bread roll (approx. 50g/2oz), plus 1 × 150g (5oz) diet yogurt

OR

4 brown Ryvitas thinly spread with low-fat soft cheese and topped with sliced tomatoes, cucumber and finely chopped lettuce

DINNER

STIR-FRIED CHICKEN AND VEGETABLES (see recipe, page 183)
PLUS
PEARS IN RED WINE (see recipe, page 180)

OR

OVEN CHIPS
(see recipe, page 179) served with dry-fried egg; broccoli and carrots
PLUS
175g (6oz) fresh fruit salad

Earlier today we touched on the fact that other members of your family may also have goals. If you and they are to succeed, these goals must not be conflicting. There is little point in your setting your heart on sailing single-handedly round the world if your other half is totally opposed to the idea! But, seriously, you do need the cooperation of your family if you are aiming for something very ambitious, because we all need support and encouragement when things get tough. Equally, the joy that can be experienced together in achieving our goals is immeasurable. You will find qualities in each other you didn't know existed.

Only one more day to go before the end of Week 3. By now I hope that you are accustomed to the pattern of eating and are finding the variety and quantities adequate to satisfy your tastebuds and appetite. Remember to be as active as possible tomorrow. Tomorrow's main meal will be at lunchtime again, so please try to prepare for it today.

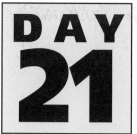

DAY 21

The last day of Week 3 — did you wonder whether you would ever get this far? Today is particularly important because it marks the three-quarter stage of a very significant goal achievement. Have you decided what your next main goal will be? Start thinking about it seriously, because in just 7 days you will be free to concentrate fully on it. You may still want to lose more weight and inches, and your top priority may be to achieve a much slimmer body than you have so far. That's fine, but you now know this will happen, and you know how to do it – just by carrying on with this New Inch Loss Plan diet and exercise programme which will have the effect of continually improving your shape.

So busy yourself today and remember, making a really special effort today could mean even more success with the tape measure and scales tomorrow morning. Stick with it and please don't cheat once today!

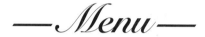

—Menu—

BREAKFAST

200g (7oz) tinned tomatoes and 115g (4oz) baked beans served on 25g (1oz) wholemeal toast

OR

2 bananas mashed with 1 × 150g (5oz) raspberry diet yogurt

LUNCH

175g (6oz) lamb's liver braised in onions, served with 50g (2oz) potatoes and unlimited other vegetables
PLUS
225g (8oz) fresh fruit

OR

SPICED BEAN CASSEROLE (see recipe, page 183)
PLUS
115g (4oz) fresh fruit and 1 × 150g (5oz) diet yogurt

SUPPER

115g (4oz) chicken (no skin) served with a large salad dressed with soy sauce, plus 1 pear and 1 banana

OR

Jacket potato (approx. 175g/6oz) topped with 75g (3oz) low-fat cottage cheese
mixed with herbs and 50g (2oz) sweetcorn, plus
BAKED STUFFED APPLE (see recipe, page 174)

WARM UP – MOBILITY AND PULSE-RAISING

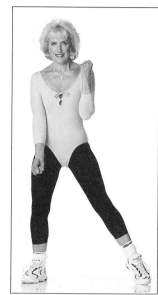

1 Step Touch with Bicep Curls Stand tall and step out to alternate sides, bending your knees as the feet come together. At the same time bend alternate elbows, keeping them close to the waist. Perform 16 times altogether.

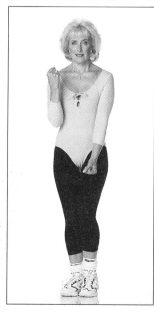

2 Squats with Arms

With feet apart, bend from the knees, letting your hips dip back as if you were trying to sit in a chair. At the same time, draw your arms straight up in front of you to shoulder height. Look straight ahead, keeping your back flat and your tummy pulled in tight against your spine. Do 8 altogether.

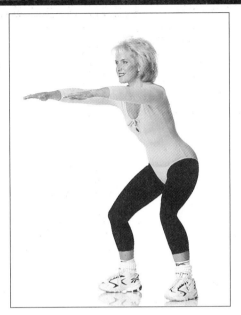

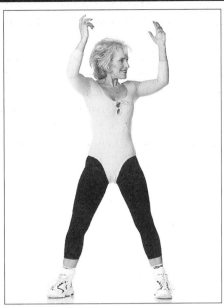

◀ **3 Waist Twists** Stand with feet apart, tummy pulled in tight and knees slightly bent. Bring your arms up to shoulder height as shown, then twist to alternate sides from the waist, keeping your hips still. Do 8 repetitions slowly and under control.

4 Half Jacks with Arms

Stand in a good posture and take the right foot out to the side, touching the floor with just the toe. At the same time lift both arms to just above shoulder height. Bring the feet together and repeat to the other side. Repeat 16 times.

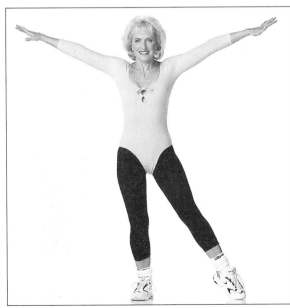

▶ **5 March on the Spot with Shoulder Lifts** Stand up straight, with your head up and your shoulders back, and march on the spot. As you march, lift both shoulders up towards your ears and then down again, keeping the action slow and controlled. Lift the shoulders for 2 marches and then lower them for 2 to keep a rhythmical pace. Lift and lower the shoulders 8 times altogether.

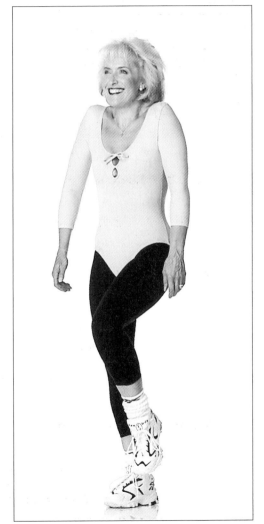

6 Calf Stretch
Stand upright, with one foot in front of the other. Keep the back leg straight and bend the front leg and make sure both feet point forward. Lean towards the front leg to feel a stretch in the lower leg at the back. Now try to take the back leg further back to gain a more effective stretch. Hold for 8 seconds, then change legs and repeat.

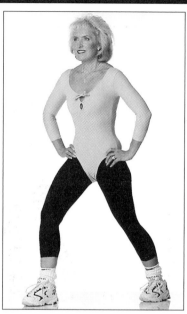

7 Lower Calf and Chest Stretch Place your right leg slightly behind the left leg and bend both knees. Keep both heels firmly on the floor and keep the hips tucked under to feel a stretch further down the calf on the right leg. Now take both hands and either clasp them behind you or place them in the small of your back and squeeze your shoulders back to feel a stretch across your chest. Keep your head up and your back straight at all times. Hold for 8 seconds, then release.

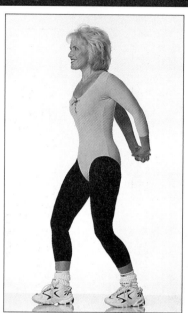

8 Lower Calf and Upper Back Stretch Place the left leg slightly behind the right leg and bend both knees. Keep both heels firmly on the floor and keep the hips tucked under to feel a stretch in the lower left leg. Now bring both arms round in front at chest height, drop your head forward and press your arms away from your upper back to feel a stretch in the upper back. Hold for 8 seconds, then release.

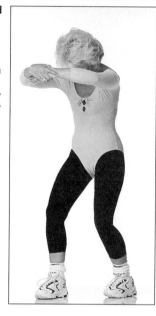

9 Back of Thigh Stretch Stand with your back leg bent and your front leg straight, and place your hands in the middle of your thighs. Now, keeping your head up and your back flat, lean forward until you feel a stretch in the back of the straight leg. Hold for 8 seconds, then change legs and repeat.

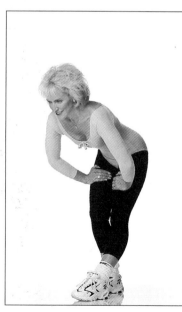

10 Front of Thigh Stretch Stand up straight and take hold around one ankle so that the knee points towards the floor and the knees are fairly close together. Try to keep the knee of the supporting leg slightly bent and push the hip forward on the held leg to feel the stretch down the front of the thigh. Hold for 8 seconds, then change legs and repeat.

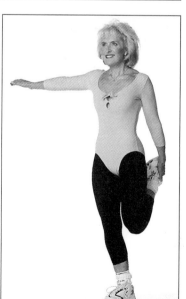

11 Tricep Stretch Stand with feet apart, tummy pulled in tight and knees slightly bent. Take your right hand behind the right shoulder and use the left hand on the fleshy part of the right underarm to push it further back. Keep your head up throughout and hold for 8 seconds. Change arms and repeat.

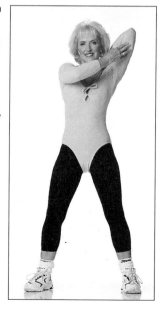

SEQUENCE 1

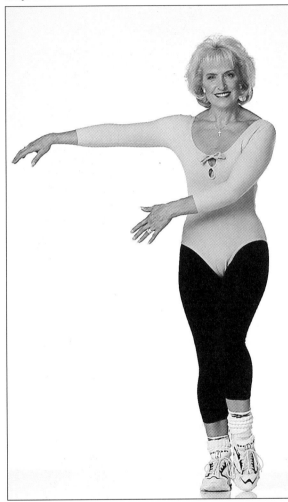

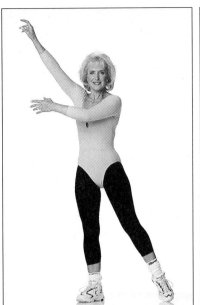

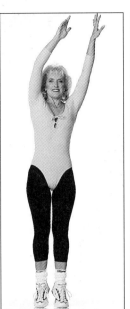

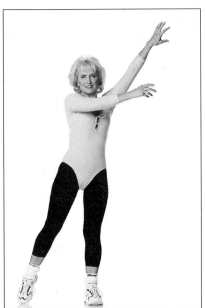

▲**12b Travel Overs** Take the 2 steps to the side, swinging your arms over in the direction that you are moving. You should now be able to add a small jump as the feet come together in the middle, but make sure your heels land on the floor if you add this. Repeat twice to each side before moving on to 12c.

12c Touch Backs As you come back from the final travel over, take the right leg back to touch the floor with the toe, leaning forward slightly and pushing your arms out in front at the same time. Do 8 touch backs with alternate legs before moving on to Sequence 2.

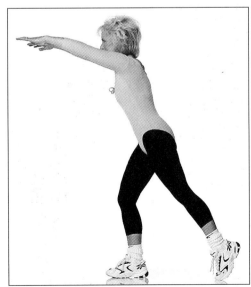

12a Step Touch Swing Step from side to side swinging the arms to just above shoulder height. Try to take wider steps now, with a deeper bend of the knees, but make sure you control the move and keep your head up and back straight. Repeat 8 times before moving on to 12b.

SEQUENCE 2

13a Hopscotch with Elbow Presses Take a step out to the side on the right leg and bend the left leg up behind. At the same time have your elbows up at shoulder height and, as the leg lifts at the back, press the elbows behind you, then repeat to the other side. Now make the steps wider and use the arms more strongly to make the move more effective. Do 8 times to alternate sides, then change to 13b.

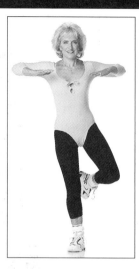

13b Walks with Rolling Arms Take 3 steps forward then clap, bringing the feet together on the 4th count, then take 3 steps back again. Roll the arms at chest height as you walk and now try to cover a lot more floor and keep tall. Repeat forward and back twice before moving on to 13c.

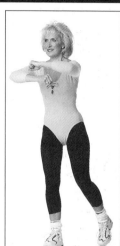

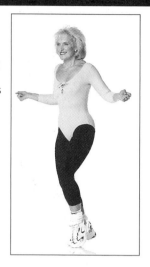

13c Skip Turns Take 4 counts to turn all the way round with a light skip, then go round the other way. Make sure the heels make contact with the floor and keep the trunk upright. Now move on to Sequence 3.

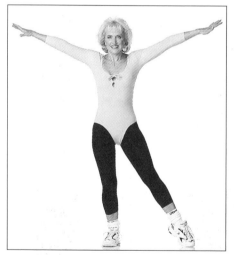

SEQUENCE 3

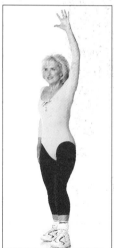

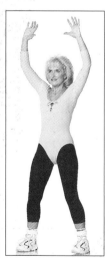

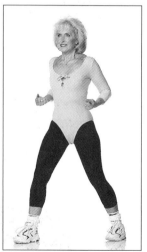

14a Box Step with High Arms Take a step forward with the right leg, leading with the heel, with the right arm overhead. Now do the same on the left side. As you step back with alternate legs, draw your elbows behind you at waist height with 2 little pushes. Step wide and use the arms strongly but keep your body upright. Do 4 box steps before moving on to 14b.

14b Half Jacks with Arms Take alternate toes out to the sides, bringing your arms out to just above shoulder height at the same time. As you change from one foot to the other add a small spring to increase the intensity of the move. Repeat 8 times under control before moving on to 14c.

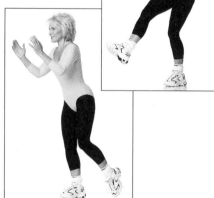

14c Double Scoops with Claps On the last half jack, turn to your right and make a scooping action with both arms as you lead off with the heel of the right foot, bringing the left foot close up behind you. Take another scoop to the right, adding a clap at the end before turning to go left. Repeat a double scoop to each side again before moving on to Sequence 4.

SEQUENCE 4

15a Grapevine with Arm Circles Take a grapevine to your right and as the feet come together at the end take 2 knee bends with a little jump off the floor, circling the arms in front of you at the same time. Now take a grapevine back to the left with 2 knee bends and arm circles on the end. Repeat twice through before moving on to 15b.

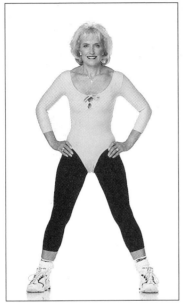

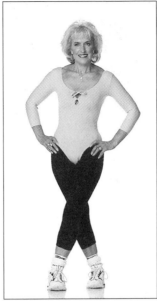

15b Alternate Squats with Jumps Next take a large squat step out to the right, really bending your knees and taking your hips back. As you come up again bring the feet together and do 2 small jumps with claps. Now do exactly the same out to the left. Keep your head up and your back straight all the time. Repeat 4 times altogether before starting again from Sequence 1.

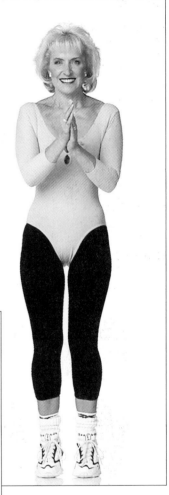

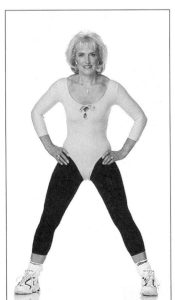

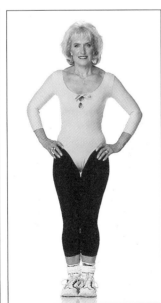

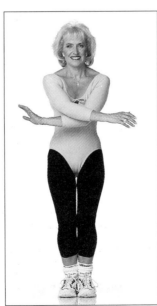

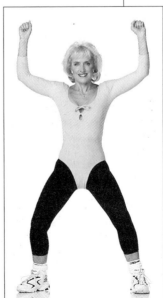

Keep repeating the sequences from 1–4 until you feel you have done enough to challenge yourself.

16 Press Ups Position yourself on your hands and knees, still using a towel under the knees if you wish. Check that your hands are directly under your shoulders and that your knees are under your hips.

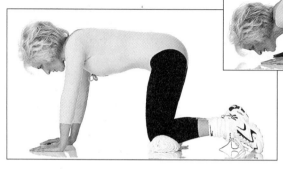

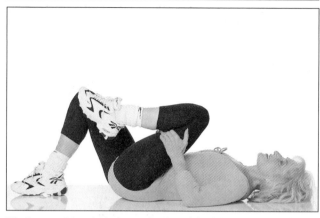

Lower your forehead down in front of your hands, then come up again without locking out the elbows. Keep your tummy pulled in and your back flat. Do 8 repetitions, then rest and repeat.

17 Back Strengthener Lie on your front, with both arms down at your sides. Keep looking at the floor and keep both feet firmly on the floor, as you gently lift your upper body off the floor. If you find this too difficult, go back to having your elbows close to your waist and the palms up in front. Do 4 repetitions, then rest and repeat.

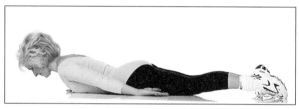

18 Bottom Toner Come up onto your forearms and knees, and place a towel under the knees if it helps. Pull your tummy in tightly and extend one leg out behind you with the toe on the floor. Now lift the leg under control to just above hip height and then lower it again. Keep both hips facing the floor and take care not to swing the leg. Do 12 repetitions, then change legs and repeat.

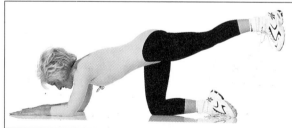

19 Abdominal Curl Lie on your back, with your knees bent and your feet flat on the floor. Place your hands at the sides of your head to support your neck (or continue to use a towel if you prefer). Now pull your tummy in towards your spine and hold it in as you lift just the head and shoulders off the floor, then lower them again. Breathe out as you lift, and breathe in as you lower. Repeat 6 times slowly, then rest and repeat.

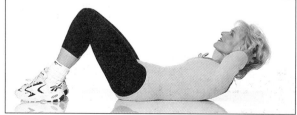

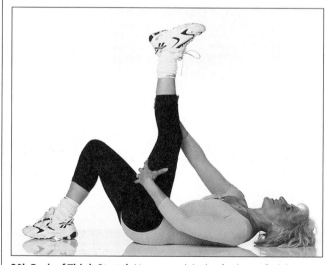

20a Bottom Stretch Lie on your back, with both knees bent and feet flat on the floor. Draw one knee into the chest, holding underneath the knee, and squeeze the raised leg towards the chest to feel a stretch in your bottom. Hold for 10 seconds, then move on to 20b.

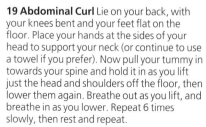

20b Back of Thigh Stretch Now extend the leg further to feel the stretch move to the back of the thigh. Keep your hips on the floor and move one hand further up the leg for support. Hold for 10 seconds, then try to extend the knee a little further in order to develop the stretch more. Hold for a further 10 seconds, then release.

Repeat 20a and 20b on the other leg.

21 Chest Stretch
Sit upright with legs still crossed. Place your hands in the small of your back and gently ease your shoulders back to feel a stretch across your chest. Hold for 8 seconds, then release.

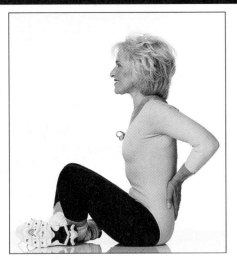

22 Spine Stretch
Sitting with legs comfortably crossed, place your hands in front of you on the floor. Lower your head and slide the hands further along the floor to feel a stretch along your spine. Hold for 8 seconds, then release.

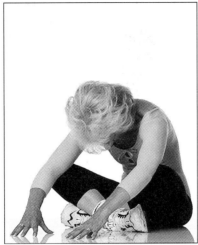

23 Abdominal Stretch
Lie on your front, place your bent arms in front of you and prop yourself up on your elbows, keeping the whole of each forearm on the floor. Now gently lift the chin forward slightly to feel a stretch down the front of the trunk. Hold for 6 seconds, then rest.

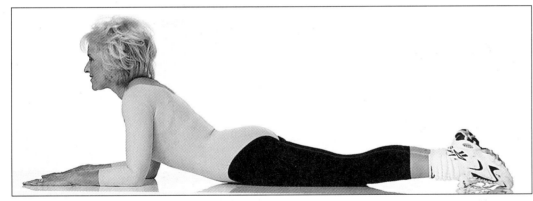

24 Front of Thigh Stretch
Lying on your front, bend your right knee up and take hold of the ankle. Ease the heel close to the hip and push that hip firmly into the floor. Hold for 10 seconds, then change legs and repeat.

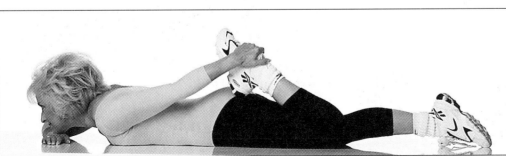

POSITIVE THOUGHT FOR THE DAY

Previously we talked about the need to want your goal – whatever that goal might be – badly enough. In other words, are you prepared to be totally persistent?

Persistence is a wonderful thing. My husband, Mike, and I used to have three cats – a mother cat and her two sons, Oscar and Harry. Oscar was quite slim and small but very streetwise. Nothing frightened him. He even attempted to take bones out of the mouths of our two German Shepherd dogs, Nikki and Sheba. He never took no for an answer. He knew exactly what he wanted and went for it, no matter what! When a neighbour's dog visited us one day, the other two cats ran away immediately. But Oscar just stood there! The visiting dog was so amazed he walked off and left Oscar alone. If you have persistence and courage, you can't fail to win, and Oscar was one of the most convincing winners I have ever met.

Please be strong tonight. Don't give in to temptation. It's weighing and measuring day tomorrow. Best of luck!

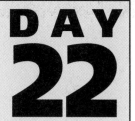

DAY 22

Did you look good when you looked in the mirror this morning? After visiting the bathroom, please measure yourself before eating or drinking anything. Then weigh yourself and record your progress.

I have designed a special celebration menu for you today. Spoil yourself with an extra drink if you wish. At each mealtime, eat enough to satisfy your appetite, even if it means having second helpings of vegetables. Better to do that, than being tempted by biscuits or sweets later.

This week your exercise time goes up to 30 minutes. You are now working hard enough and long enough for them to be really effective. Well done!.

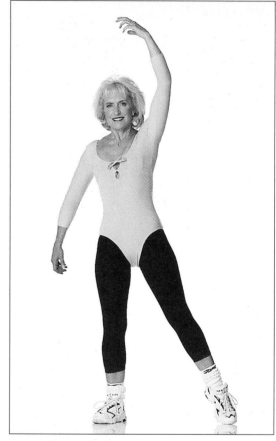

1 Weight Transfer with Arm Circles Transfer your weight from one foot to the other and at the same time take the opposite arm in a circling action just above the head. So, as you take the weight to the right leg, the left arm goes over and so on. Control the move and pull your tummy in and maintain a good posture. Repeat 16 times altogether.

—Menu—

BREAKFAST

25g (1oz) lean ham served with 2 tomatoes and 1 wholemeal roll spread (approx. 50g/2oz) with mustard or pickle

OR

25g (1oz) any cereal and 115g (4oz) sliced fruit of your choice, served with milk from allowance and 1 teaspoon of sugar

LUNCH

4 slices of light bread (max. 200kcals) spread with SEAFOOD DRESSING (see recipe, page 182) and filled with salad and 115g (4oz) prawns, plus 75g (3oz) low-fat fromage frais

OR

Large bowl (250ml/8fl oz) vegetable soup with 1 wholemeal bap (approx. 50g/2oz), plus 1 × 150g (5oz) diet yogurt

DINNER

SPAGHETTI BOLOGNESE (see recipe, page 182)
PLUS
PINEAPPLE BOAT (see recipe, page 180)

OR

VEGETARIAN SPAGHETTI BOLOGNESE (see recipe, page 185)
PLUS
OATY YOGURT DESSERT (see recipe, page 179)

Plus an extra glass of wine to celebrate completion of your third week!

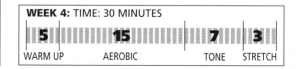

WEEK 4: TIME: 30 MINUTES

5	15	7	3
WARM UP	AEROBIC	TONE	STRETCH

2 Side Bends with Twists

2a Standing with feet apart, shoulders back and head up, lean slightly to the right, reaching your right arm out and lifting the left elbow up. Come up and lean to the other side. Do 4 repetitions, then change to 2b.

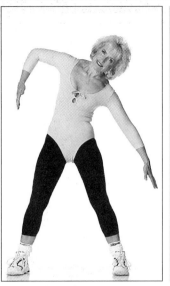

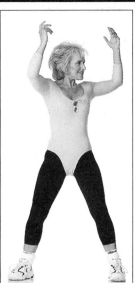

2b Bring the arms up in line with the shoulders as shown and, keeping your hips facing forward, twist the upper body round to the right. Come back to face front and repeat to the left. Do 4 repetitions and then repeat 2a and 2b once more.

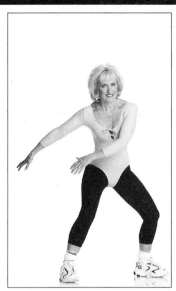

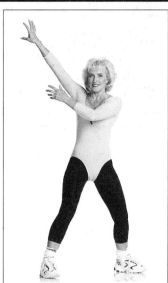

4 Twisted Heel/Toe

Take the right heel diagonally out in front on the floor. Keep it there as you twist from the hip and change to the toe. Alternate from heel to toe to a count of 8 then repeat to the left side.

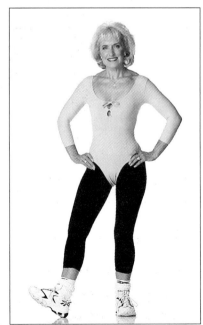

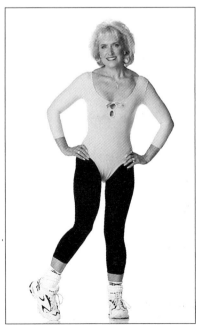

3 Squats with Figure of 8 Arms Stand with feet apart and take a rhythmical squat, making sure the knees bend in the direction of the toes. At the same time make a figure of 8 with your arms in front of you. Do 16 altogether.

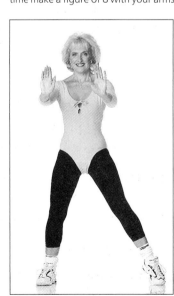

5 Double Steps with Arm Presses

Take 2 steps to the right and, at the same time, press both arms out in front at chest height. Now take 2 steps back to the left. Keep your body upright, with your shoulders back and your head up. Repeat the sequence 4 times altogether.

6 Inner Thigh and Waist Stretch
Stand with feet wide apart, and start with an inner thigh stretch by bending your right knee in line with the toes and keeping the left leg straight, with the foot pointing forward. Feel the stretch in the inner thigh. Now take your left arm up over your head and lean slightly to the right to feel the stretch in your waist. Hold for 8 seconds, then repeat to the other side.

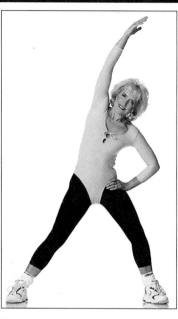

7 Front of Thigh Stretch Stand up straight and take hold around one ankle so that the knee points towards the floor and the knees are fairly close together. Try to keep the knee of the supporting leg slightly bent and push the hip forward on the held leg to feel the stretch down the front of the thigh. Hold for 8 seconds, then change legs and repeat.

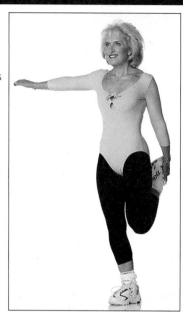

8 Calf Stretch
Stand upright, with one foot in front of the other. Keep the back leg straight and bend the front leg and make sure both feet point forward. Lean towards the front leg to feel a stretch in the lower leg at the back. Now try to take the back leg further back to gain a more effective stretch. Hold for 8 seconds, then change legs and repeat.

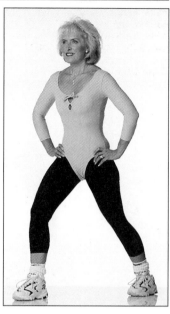

9 Lower Calf and Chest Stretch Place your right leg slightly behind the left leg and bend both knees. Keep both heels firmly on the floor and keep the hips tucked under to feel a stretch further down the calf on the right leg. Now take both hands and either clasp them behind you or place them in the small of your back and squeeze your shoulders back to feel a stretch across your chest. Keep your head up and your back straight at all times. Hold for 8 seconds, then release.

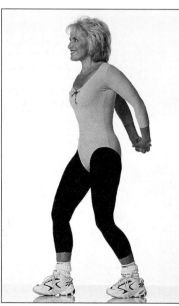

10 Lower Calf and Upper Back Stretch Place the left leg slightly behind the right leg and bend both knees. Keep both heels firmly on the floor and keep the hips tucked under to feel a stretch in the lower left leg. Now bring both arms round in front at chest height, drop your head forward and press your arms away from your upper back to feel a stretch in the upper back. Hold for 8 seconds, then release.

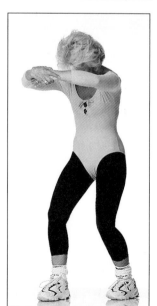

11 Back of Thigh Stretch Stand with your back leg bent and your front leg straight, and place your hands in the middle of your thighs. Now, keeping your head up and your back flat, lean forward until you feel a stretch in the back of the straight leg. Hold for 8 seconds, then change legs and repeat.

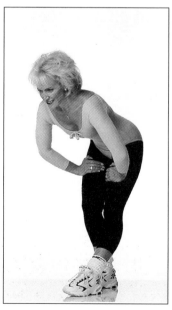

You should continue to increase the amount of time you spend on this session, as the more you can do, the more effectively you will attack those fat stores and lose those inches. Only do as much as is right for you. Generally speaking, you should be able to keep going for the whole 15 minutes, but you might need to work at a lower level by keeping the arms below shoulder level or not using them at all, and by avoiding any jumping which considerably increases the intensity. This week you are encouraged to jump more, but make sure this only occurs in the *middle* of this session and not at the beginning or end, so that you allow the pulse rate to raise and lower safely.

SEQUENCE 1

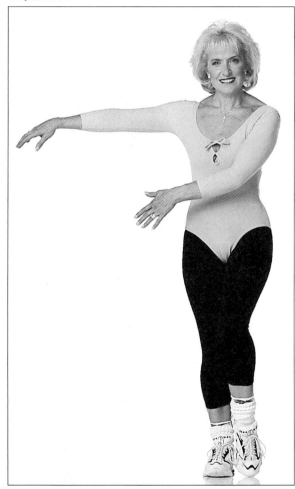

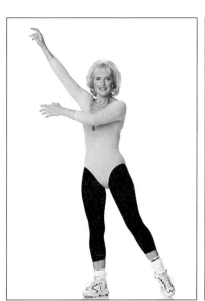

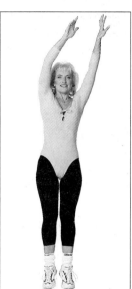

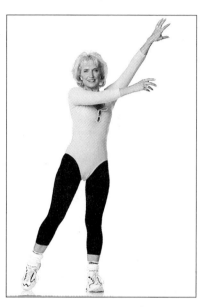

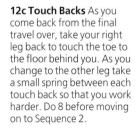

▲ 12b Travel Overs Take 2 steps to the side, swinging your arms over in the direction you are moving. Add a little jump as the feet come together, making sure both heels land on the floor each time. Repeat twice to each side before moving on to 12c.

12c Touch Backs As you come back from the final travel over, take your right leg back to touch the toe to the floor behind you. As you change to the other leg take a small spring between each touch back so that you work harder. Do 8 before moving on to Sequence 2.

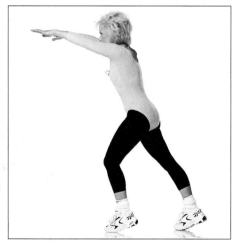

12a Step Touch Swing Step from side to side, swinging your arms above shoulder height. Keep the move controlled and keep your head up and your shoulders well back, but try to work really hard with each step. Do 8 before changing to 12b.

SEQUENCE 2

13a Hopscotch with High Arms Take a step out to the side on the right leg, taking your arms high above your head. Now, as you bend the left leg up behind draw the arms strongly down by your sides to finish the move. Change to the other side and keep alternating sides for 8 repetitions before moving on to 13b.

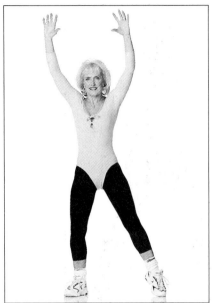

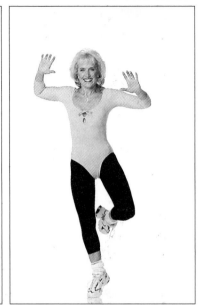

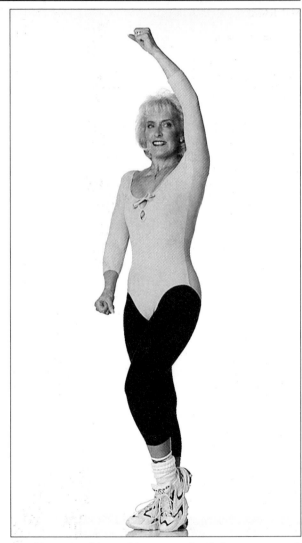

13b Walks with Rolling Arms Take 3 steps forward, then bring the feet together with a jump and a clap on the 4th count. Repeat moving backwards. Roll the arms at chest height as you travel and aim to cover more ground and take bigger jumps as the routine progresses. Repeat forward and back twice before moving on to 13c.

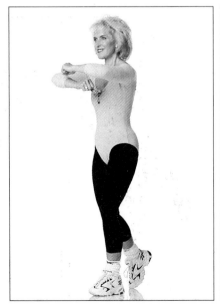

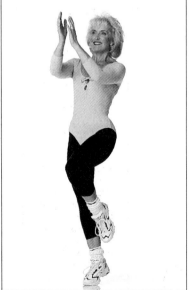

13c Skip Turns with Punching Arms Take 4 full counts to turn all the way round with a jumping skip, really lifting the knees now, and punch alternate arms up in the air as you skip. Then go back the other way. Check the heels land on the floor each time you skip, control the arm movement and keep tall. Now move on to Sequence 3.

SEQUENCE 3

14a Box Step with High Arms Take a step forward with the right leg, leading with the heel, with the right arm overhead. As you step back with alternate legs, draw your elbows behind you at waist height with 2 little pushes. Step wide and use the arms strongly but keep your body upright. Do 4 box steps before moving on to 14b.

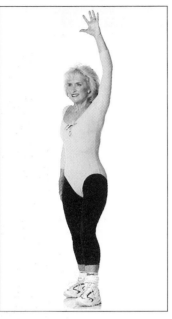
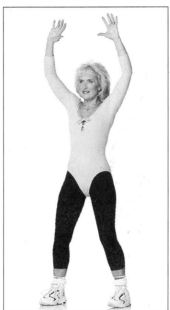
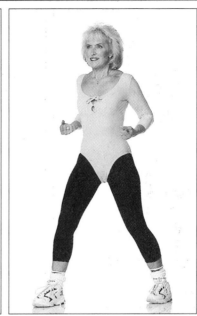

14b Half Jacks with Arms Take alternate toes out to the sides, bringing your arms out to just above shoulder height at the same time. As you change from one foot to the other add a small spring to increase the intensity of the move. Repeat 8 times under control before moving on to 14c.

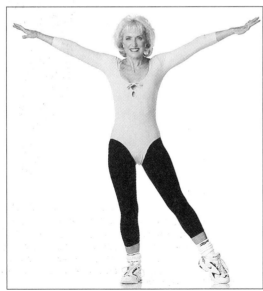

14c Double Scoops with Claps On the last half jack, turn to your right and make a scooping action with both arms as you lead off with the heel of the right foot, bringing the left foot up close behind. Take another scoop to the right, adding a clap and a jump before turning to go left. Repeat a double scoop to each side before moving on to Sequence 4.

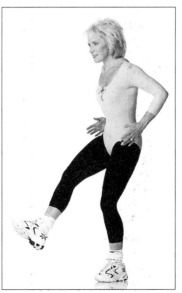
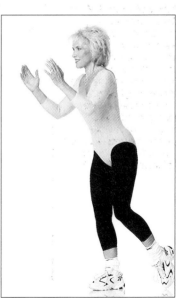

SEQUENCE 4

15a Grapevine with Arm Circles

Take a grapevine to your right and as the feet come together at the end take 2 knee bends with a little jump off the floor, circling the arms at the same time. Now take a grapevine back to the left with 2 knee bends and arm circles on the end. Repeat twice through before moving on to 15b.

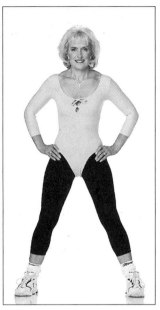
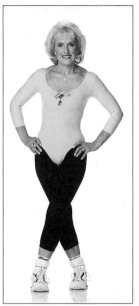
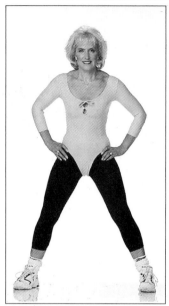
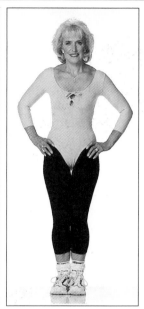
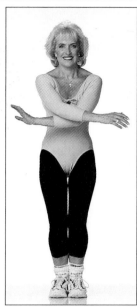

15b Alternate Squats with Jumps

Next take a large squat step out to the right, really bending your knees and taking your hips back. As you come up again bring the feet together and do 2 small jumps with claps. Now do exactly the same out to the left. Keep your head up and your back straight all the time. Repeat 4 times altogether before moving on to 15c.

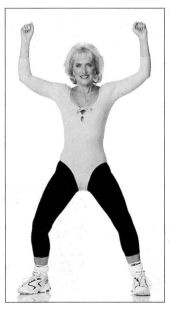
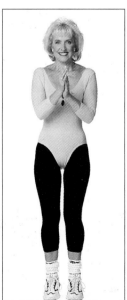
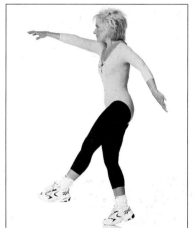
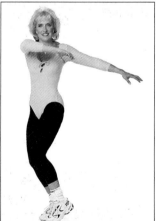

15c Kick Away Forward and Twist Back

Take a step forward on the right foot and continue to travel forward as you kick the left leg forward. Keep alternating legs, travelling forward until you have completed 4 kicks. Now twist backwards for 4 counts. Stand tall throughout and make sure those heels go down as you land. Repeat twice through before going back to Sequence 1.

Keep repeating the sequences for as long as suits you, hopefully building up to the full 15 minutes by the end of the week, making sure you work hard enough to become slightly breathless and very warm. Enjoy it!

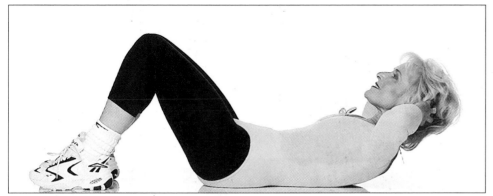

16 Abdominal Curl Lie on your back, with your knees bent and your feet flat on the floor. Place your hands at the sides of your head to support your neck (or continue to use a towel if you prefer). Now pull your tummy in towards your spine and hold it in as you lift just the head and shoulders off the floor, then lower them again. Breathe out as you lift, and breathe in as you lower. Repeat 8 times slowly, then rest and repeat.

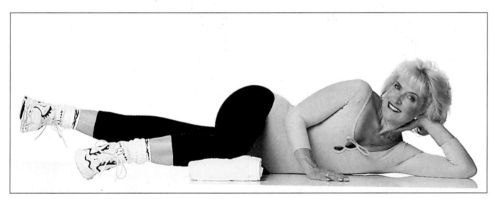

17 Inner Thigh Toner Lie on your side and place the top leg over the underneath leg, still using the towel under the knee for extra comfort if you wish. Smoothly lift the underneath leg, then lower it again. Repeat 16 times, then rest and repeat. Roll over and repeat with the other leg.

▼ **19 Bottom Toner** Come up onto your forearms and knees, and place a towel under the knees if you wish. Pull your tummy in tightly and extend one leg out behind you with the toe on the floor. Now lift the leg under control to just above hip height and then lower it again. Keep both hips facing the floor and take care not to swing the leg. Do 16 repetitions, then change legs and repeat.

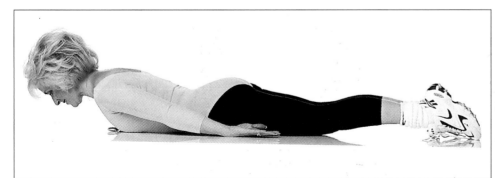

18 Back Strengthener Lie on your front, with both arms down at your sides. Keep looking at the floor and keep both feet firmly on the floor, as you gently lift your upper body off the floor. Do 6 repetitions, then rest and repeat.

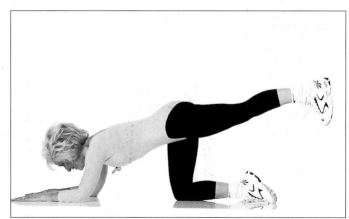

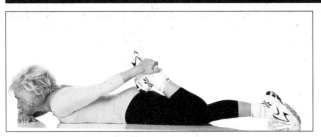

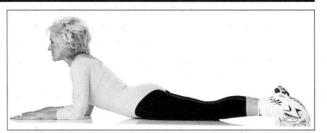

20 Front of Thigh Stretch Lie on your front, bend your right knee up and take hold of the ankle. Ease the heel close to the hip and push that hip firmly into the floor. Hold for 10 seconds, then change legs and repeat.

21 Abdominal Stretch Lying on your front, place your bent arms in front of you and prop yourself up on your elbows, keeping the whole of each forearm on the floor. Now gently lift the chin forward slightly to feel a stretch down the front of the trunk. Hold for 6 seconds, then rest.

22 Spine Stretch Sit with legs comfortably crossed and place your hands in front of you on the floor. Lower your head and slide the hands further along the floor to feel a stretch along your spine. Hold for 8 seconds, then release.

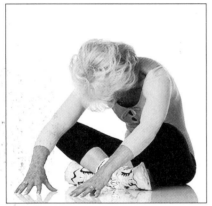

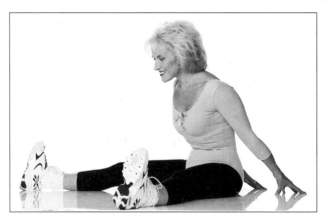

23 Inner Thigh Stretch Sit with your legs comfortably wide apart, and lift up tall, with your back straight and your head up. Place your hands behind your hips and use them to help you push your pelvis further forward. Now lean forward, still keeping your back straight, and feel a strong stretch in the inner thighs. (If this does not suit you, you can return to the easier version of this stretch with soles of the feet together.) Hold for 10 seconds, then take a deep breath in and, as you breathe out, lean further forward to hold for another 10 seconds.

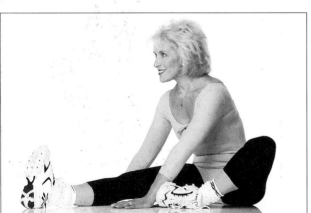

24 Back of Thigh Stretch Sit up, with one leg diagonally out in front of you and the other leg tucked up in front of the hip as shown. Place your hands to either side of the straight leg and, keeping your back flat and your head up, lean forward slightly to feel a stretch in the back of the thigh. Hold for 10 seconds, then try to lean even further forward, without bending the spine, to develop the stretch more, and hold for a further 10 seconds. Change legs and repeat.

POSITIVE THOUGHT FOR THE DAY

Have you enjoyed your special day, or didn't anyone notice your terrific new image? Just because no one said anything doesn't mean that your progress went unnoticed. People can be very shy about giving compliments. While it is true that we shouldn't 'show off' our new slim figure, there's nothing wrong in making the most of it.

Complimenting people is a real pleasure – as much for the recipient as for the person giving it. When did you last tell your partner that you find him or her very attractive? That you still fancy him or her. That you really love them. That you appreciate all that they do for you, their consideration, their thoughtfulness etc. I have no doubt there are many things you wish they didn't do, or were not, but there must be some good points! If there are, say which they are instead of pointing out only the faults. This also applies to children, employees and even employers. No one is above a compliment. Try it and see what happens. I promise it will make for a more positive atmosphere around you.

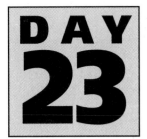

DAY 23

Today I would like you to consciously attempt to reduce the negative elements in your life. I have often described this philosophy as preparing a garden full of flowers by removing all the weeds. This has the effect of eliminating from our daily lives all those negative influences, problems and restrictions and replacing them with the seeds of positive plans, happiness and an expansive and creative mind.

There is no doubt that we are influenced by those around us and by our parents throughout childhood. Many an adult struggles with their weight because of being persuaded to 'eat up' as a child. In our minds 'eating everything that is placed in front of us' is associated with 'well done, that's a nice clean plate'. All kinds of conditioning causes us to act in a way that we know is contrary to what we really want. So try and be strong in your decisions and don't accept past conditioning as being 'the law'.

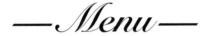

— *Menu* —

BREAKFAST

3 figs and 1 × 150g (5oz) diet yogurt, any flavour

OR

1 scrambled egg on 25g (1oz) toast with 2 grilled tomatoes

LUNCH

115g (4oz) mackerel or tuna (in brine) served with a large chopped salad and 2 tablespoons reduced-oil salad dressing, plus 1 × 150g (5oz) diet yogurt

OR

4 Ryvitas spread with low-fat soft cheese and topped with low-calorie coleslaw and sliced tomatoes, plus 1 piece of fresh fruit

DINNER

FISH CURRY (see recipe, page 176)
PLUS
PEARS IN MERINGUE (see recipe, page 180)

OR

VEGETABLE CURRY (see recipe, page 184)
PLUS
PINEAPPLE IN KIRSCH (see recipe, page 180)

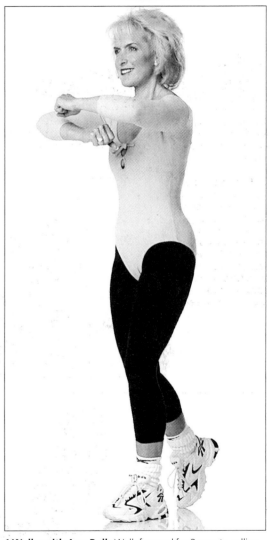

1 Walks with Arm Rolls Walk forward for 3 counts, rolling the arms at chest height, and on the 4th count bring the feet together and clap, then walk backwards again and clap. Stand tall, with your head up and your tummy pulled in. Move forward and back 4 times altogether.

2 Side Bends with Twists 2a Standing with feet apart, shoulders back and head up, lean slightly to the right, reaching your right arm out and lifting the left elbow up. Come up and lean to the other side. Do 4 repetitions, then change to 2b.

2b Bring the arms up in line with the shoulders as shown and, keeping your hips facing forward, twist the upper body round to the right. Come back to face front and repeat to the left. Do 4 repetitions and then repeat 2a and 2b once more.

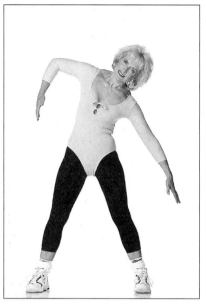 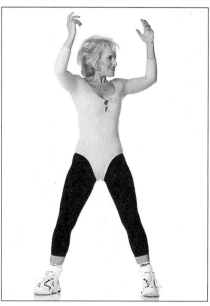

3 Side Steps with Monkey Arms Take 2 steps out to the right, with your arms straight out in front, pulling them up and down alternately in rhythm with the steps. Take 2 steps back to the left and keep going, to repeat the sequence 4 times altogether.

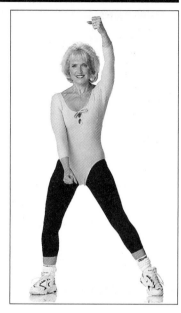

4 Weight Transfer with Arm Circles
Transfer your weight from one foot to the other and at the same time take the opposite arm in a circling action just above the head. So, as you take the weight to the right leg, the left arm goes over and so on. Control the move and pull your tummy in and maintain a good posture. Repeat 16 times altogether.

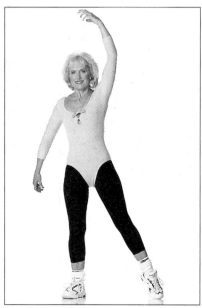

5 Ski Swings Stand with feet together and lift your arms above your head. Pulling your tummy in tight and keeping your head up, swing down, bending your knees and taking the arms behind you as shown. Lift and lower under control 6 times altogether.

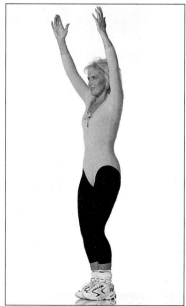 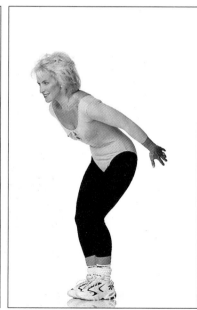

6 Inner Thigh and Waist Stretch

Stand with feet wide apart, and start with an inner thigh stretch by bending your right knee in line with the toes and keeping the left leg straight, with the foot pointing forward. Feel the stretch in the inner thigh. Now take your left arm up over your head and lean slightly to the right to feel the stretch in your waist. Hold for 8 seconds, then repeat to the other side.

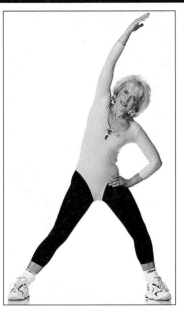

7 Calf Stretch

Stand upright, with one foot in front of the other. Keep the back leg straight and bend the front leg and make sure both feet point forward. Lean towards the front leg to feel a stretch in the lower leg at the back. Now try to take the back leg further back to gain a more effective stretch. Hold for 8 seconds, then change legs and repeat.

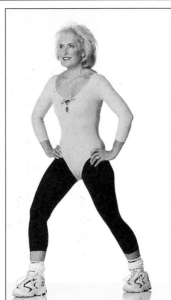

8 Lower Calf and Chest Stretch

Place your right leg slightly behind the left leg and bend both knees. Keep both heels firmly on the floor and keep the hips tucked under to feel a stretch further down the calf on the right leg. Now take both hands and either clasp them behind you or place them in the small of your back and squeeze your shoulders back to feel a stretch across your chest. Keep your head up and your back straight at all times. Hold for 8 seconds, then release.

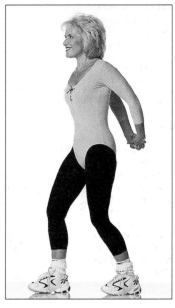

9 Lower Calf and Upper Back Stretch

Place the left leg slightly behind the right leg and bend both knees. Keep both heels firmly on the floor and keep the hips tucked under to feel a stretch in the lower left leg. Now bring both arms round in front at chest height, drop your head forward and press your arms away from your upper back to feel a stretch in the upper back. Hold for 8 seconds, then release.

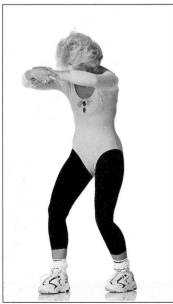

10 Front of Thigh Stretch

Stand up straight and take hold around one ankle so that the knee points towards the floor and the knees are fairly close together. Try to keep the knee of the supporting leg slightly bent and push the hip forward on the held leg to feel the stretch down the front of the thigh. Hold for 8 seconds, then change legs and repeat.

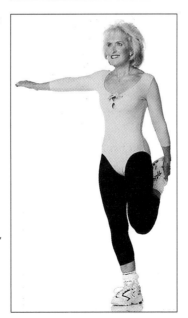

11 Back of Thigh Stretch

Stand with your back leg bent and your front leg straight, and place your hands in the middle of your thighs. Now, keeping your head up and your back flat, lean forward until you feel a stretch in the back of the straight leg. Hold for 8 seconds, then change legs and repeat.

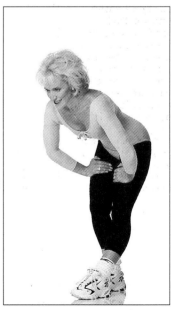

SEQUENCE 1

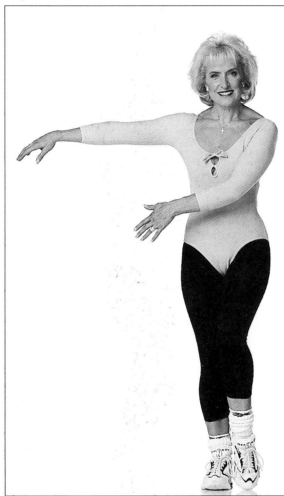

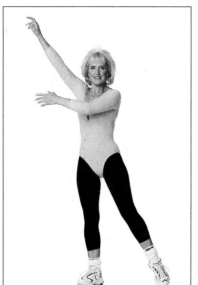 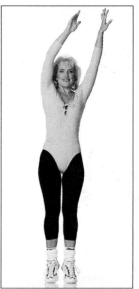 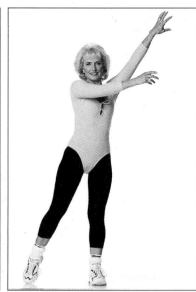

▲ **12b Travel Overs** Take 2 steps to the side, swinging your arms over in the direction you are moving. Add a little jump as the feet come together, making sure both heels land on the floor each time. Repeat twice to each side before moving on to 12c.

12c Touch Backs As you come back from the final travel over, take your right leg back to touch the toe to the floor behind you. As you change to the other leg take a small spring between each touch back so that you work harder. Do 8 before moving on to Sequence 2.

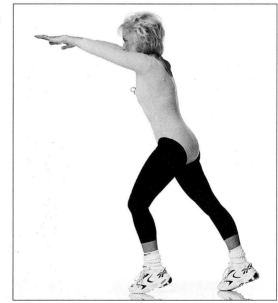

12a Step Touch Swing Step from side to side, swinging your arms above shoulder height. Keep the move controlled, with your head up and your shoulders well back, but try to work really hard with each step. Do 8 before changing to 12b.

SEQUENCE 2

13a Hopscotch with High Arms Take a step out to the side on the right leg, taking your arms high above your head. Now, as you bend the left leg up behind draw the arms strongly down by your sides to finish the move. Change to the other side and keep alternating sides for 8 repetitions before moving on to 13b.

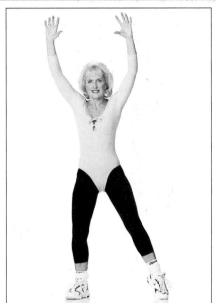

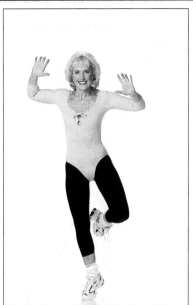

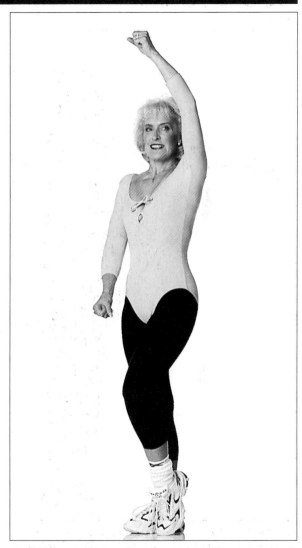

13b Walks with Rolling Arms Take 3 steps forward, then bring the feet together with a jump and a clap on the 4th count. Repeat moving backwards. Roll the arms at chest height as you travel and aim to cover more ground and take bigger jumps as the routine progresses. Repeat forward and back twice before moving on to 13c.

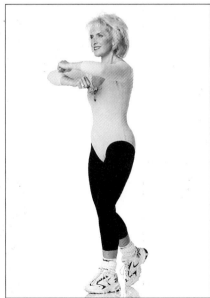

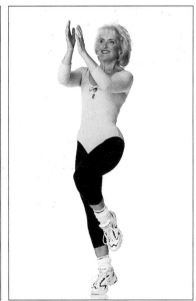

13c Skip Turns with Punching Arms Take 4 full counts to turn all the way round with a jumping skip, really lifting the knees now, and punch alternate arms up in the air as you skip. Then go back the other way. Check the heels land on the floor each time you skip, control the arm movement and keep tall. Now move on to Sequence 3.

SEQUENCE 3

14a Box Step with High Arms Take a step forward with the right leg, leading with the heel, with the right arm overhead. Now do the same on the left side. As you step back with alternate legs, draw your elbows behind you at waist height with 2 little pushes. Step wide and use the arms strongly but keep your body upright. Do 4 box steps before moving on to 14b.

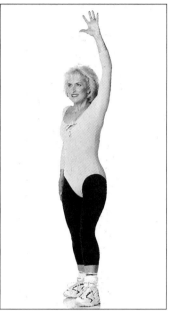 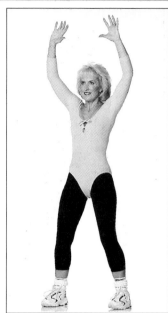 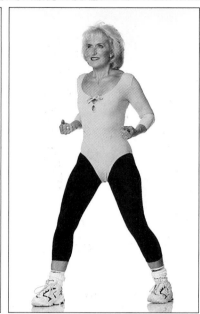

14b Half Jacks with Arms Take alternate toes out to the sides, bringing your arms out to just above shoulder height at the same time. As you change from one foot to the other add a small spring to increase the intensity of the move. Repeat 8 times under control before moving on to 14c.

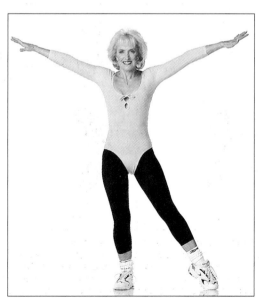

14c Double Scoops with Claps On the last half jack, turn to your right and make a scooping action with both arms as you lead off with the heel of the right foot, bringing the left foot up close behind. Take another scoop to the right, adding a clap and a jump before turning to go left. Repeat a double scoop to each side before moving on to Sequence 4.

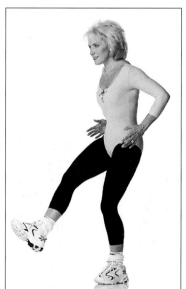 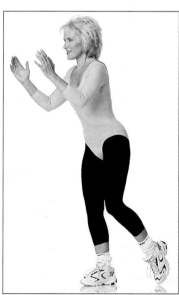

SEQUENCE 4

15a Grapevine with Arm Circles

Take a grapevine to your right and as the feet come together at the end take 2 knee bends with a little jump off the floor, circling the arms in front of you at the same time. Now take a grapevine back to the left with 2 knee bends and arm circles on the end. Repeat twice through before moving on to 15b.

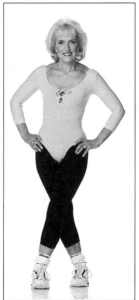 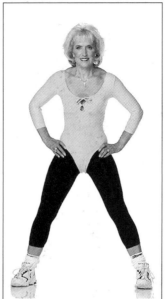 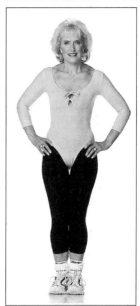 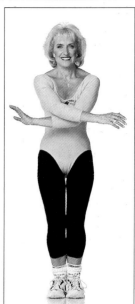

15b Alternate Squats with Jumps

Next take a large squat step out to the right, really bending your knees and taking your hips back. As you come up again bring the feet together and do 2 small jumps with claps. Now do exactly the same out to the left. Keep your head up and your back straight all the time. Repeat 4 times altogether before moving on to 15c.

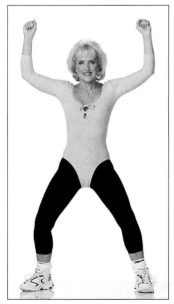 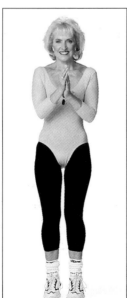

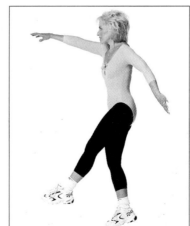 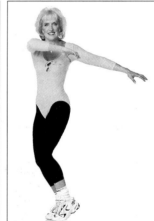

15c Kick Away Forward and Twist Back

Take a step forward on the right foot and continue to travel forward as you kick the left leg forward. Keep alternating legs, travelling forward until you have completed 4 kicks. Now twist backwards for 4 counts. Stand tall throughout and make sure those heels go down as you land. Repeat twice through before going back to Sequence 1.

Keep repeating the sequences until you feel you have worked long and hard enough to suit your ability.

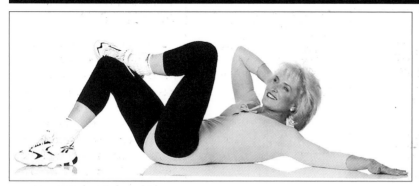

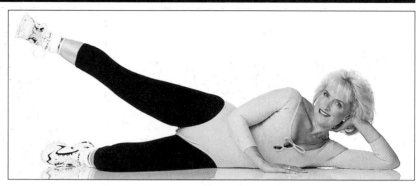

16 Waist Crunches Lie on your back, with your right leg bent and the foot flat on the floor. Now place your left ankle across the knee of the right leg, allowing the left knee to drop outwards slightly. Place your right hand behind your head for support and place your left arm out straight, at a right angle to the body. Now pull your tummy in against your spine and lift your upper body, bringing your right shoulder towards your left knee. Breathe out as you lift and in as you lower. Lift 8 times, then change sides and repeat.

17 Outer Thigh Toner Lie on your side, propped on your elbow. The underneath leg is bent and the top leg is now straight, with the hips stacked on top of each other. Now lift the top leg to just above hip height, keeping the foot pointing forward and without tipping the hips back. Lower the leg again and repeat. Do 16 repetitions, then roll over and repeat with the other leg.

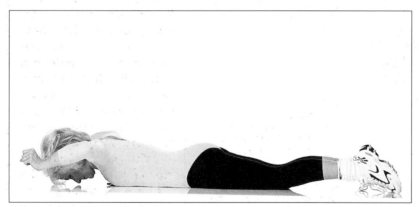

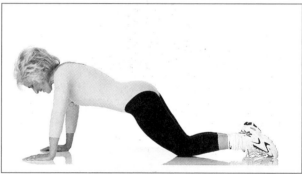

18 Posture Improver Lie down on your front and place your arms out at the sides at right angles, with the elbows at shoulder height. Keep your head in contact with the floor as you gently lift the shoulders to squeeze the shoulder blades together. Breathe out as you lift and breathe in as you go down. Keep the movement smooth. Do 4 repetitions then rest and repeat.

19 Elongated Press Ups Come up onto your hands and knees and pull your tummy in tight to flatten your back. Make sure your hands are directly underneath your shoulders but now take the knees further back as shown, to increase the weight carried by the arms. (Go back to the square box position if this is too hard.) Now lower and lift the upper body, taking care not to lock the elbows out at the top. Breathe out as you lift and breathe in as you lower. Do 6 repetitions, then rest and repeat.

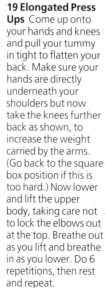

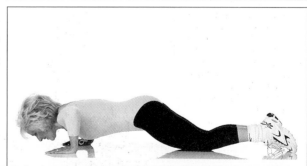

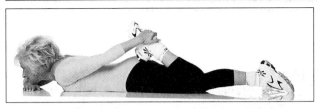

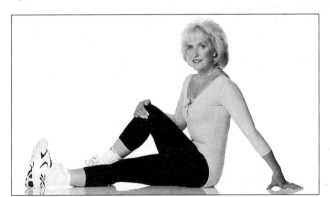

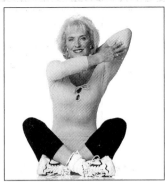

20 Front of Thigh Stretch Lie on your front, bend your right knee up and take hold of the ankle. Ease the heel close to the hip and push that hip firmly into the floor. Hold for 10 seconds, then change legs and repeat.

21 Outer Thigh Stretch Sit with both legs out in front, then cross your right leg over the left and place your right foot in line with the left knee. Now place your left hand on the outside of the right knee and the other hand on the floor for support. Gently squeeze the right knee further across the chest to feel a stretch in the outer thigh. Hold for 8 seconds, then release. Change legs and repeat.

22 Chest Stretch Sit with your legs crossed, your back straight and your head up. Take both hands behind you and clasp them loosely. Now keeping your elbows bent, squeeze your shoulders back to feel a stretch across your chest. Hold for 8 seconds, then release.

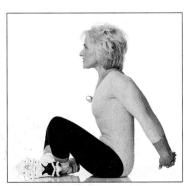

23 Tricep Stretch Sitting with legs crossed, head up and shoulders back, place your right hand behind your right shoulder and take the left hand across in front to push the arm further back. Hold for 6 seconds, then change sides and repeat.

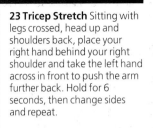

24 Upper Back Stretch Sitting cross-legged, bring both arms round in front of you at chest height and clasp your hands. Drop your head forward, and round your spine to feel a stretch across the back of the shoulders. Hold for 8 seconds, then release.

25 Waist Stretch Sit upright, with legs comfortably crossed. Lift your right arm up in the air toward the ceiling and place your left hand on the floor for support. Now, keeping both hips firmly on the floor, lean slightly to the left to feel a stretch down the waist on the right side. Hold for 8 seconds, then release and repeat to the other side.

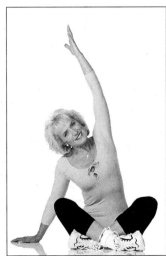

POSITIVE THOUGHT FOR THE DAY

I'd like you to consider removing from your life, one by one, all those things that annoy you, that get you down, that upset you. If you like your job but can't get on with the people with whom you have to work, consider asking for a transfer to another department. If your partner has a particular habit that annoys you, tell them about it. I bet they don't even know they're doing it!

Another way to describe these problems is to call them 'Chinese drip tortures'. In other words, little things that drive us mad. If we can remove these little stresses, or 'weeds' from our lives, it makes such a difference. But unless we communicate our desires and feelings to those who are involved, how on earth will they know?

What are the 'weeds' in your life? Start making a list and begin eliminating them, one by one. It's easier than you think.

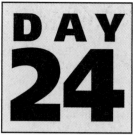

DAY 24

Are you pleased with your progress so far? Sometimes it can be slightly embarrassing to be successful at something, and if you are beginning to turn the occasional head now that you are slimmer, you may come in for some negative comments from your rivals. There will always be someone only too eager to criticise your progress. It is important to protect yourself from such killjoys.

What we can do is to choose our friends and only listen to those whose opinion we totally respect. There is nothing wrong with criticism when it is constructive. And remind yourself that you have worked very hard indeed to achieve the success you are now enjoying and you jolly well deserve it. Having a positive attitude about your progress will ensure you have continued success.

Take another break from the exercise programme today. Plan a long walk or take a bike ride instead.

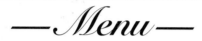

—Menu—

BREAKFAST

$^1/_2$ a fresh pineapple, chopped and mixed with 5oz (150g) pineapple diet yogurt

OR

25g (1oz) any cereal mixed with 1 × 5oz (150g) diet yogurt

LUNCH

1 slimmer's cup-a-soup, plus 2 brown Ryvitas spread with 2 teaspoons of Branston pickle and topped with 50g (2oz) wafer thin chicken or turkey, plus 115g (4oz) fresh fruit

OR

2 slices of light bread spread with Marmite and 115g (4oz) low-fat cottage cheese, served with salad, plus 1 banana

DINNER

FISH KEBABS (see recipe, page 177)
PLUS
BAKED APPLES WITH APRICOTS (see recipe, page 173)

OR

GARLIC MUSHROOMS (see recipe, page 177)
RATATOUILLE
(see recipe, page 181) served with 1 × 225g (8oz) jacket potato and unlimited other vegetables
PLUS
RASPBERRY FLUFF (see recipe, page 181)

As I have said earlier, we all need encouragement and, often, remarks from the most unexpected quarters are the most gratifying.

Pauline Singleton wrote to me regarding her success on the Hip and Thigh Diet. She managed to reduce her weight by 1st 2lb (7.2kg) in 9 weeks to a delightfully slim 8st 5lb (53.2kg) for her 5ft 5in (1.65m) height.

Pauline wrote: 'I was thrilled at how quickly and easily the inches melted away. Other diets left me feeling tired and sickly, but on this one I feel great. Neighbours and friends keep telling me I look slim. I tried to get the book for my sister-in-law for her birthday but most places were sold out. When I explained this to the assistant she said: "Oh, I didn't think the book could be for yourself – you're lovely and slim."' I bet that comment made Pauline's day. We all need to be told we look good, so try to educate your family to support you in this way.

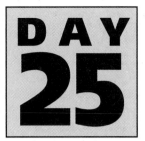

DAY 25

As you approach the end of the diet and exercise programme, it is important to decide at this stage how you intend to proceed afterwards. If you have a significant amount of weight to lose, you have the choice of continuing with the diet menus as included in the daily plans or you can follow a diet from any of my other books. The diets are similar in so far as they are all low fat, thereby maximising the reduction of fat from the body and are based on around 1,400 calories a day.

If you are almost down to your goal weight and inches you should follow the instructions in the Maintenance Programme detailed on page 000. In fact, I recommend everyone follows the Maintenance Programme for one week after finishing the 28-day programme. It will give you a break from the restrictions that have been placed upon you and will enable you to see how you manage on your own! Having a break for a week also has the benefit of jollying up the metabolism so that your body won't think you are dieting. Your weight and inches should remain constant during that week and then, when you return to the diet, you will probably find you lose weight and inches quite easily.

Some slimmers feel they need supervision and support, and there are lots of Rosemary Conley Diet & Fitness Clubs throughout the UK. All our instructors are qualified exercise teachers as well as having received comprehensive training in low-fat eating. (See the back page of this book for details.)

—Menu—

BREAKFAST
25g (1oz) bran cereal with 15g (½oz) sultanas and milk from allowance

OR

2 slices of toast with 3 teaspoons of marmalade, preserve or honey

LUNCH
CURRIED CHICKEN
AND YOGURT SALAD
(see recipe, page 176),
plus 75g (3oz) low-fat fromage frais

OR

ORANGE AND CARROT SALAD
(see recipe, page 179)
plus 2 × 150g (2 × 5oz) diet yogurts

DINNER
FISH RISOTTO
(see recipe, page 177)
PLUS
115g (4oz) fresh strawberries or raspberries served with 50g (2oz) iced yogurt

OR

BARBECUED VEGETABLE KEBABS
(see recipe, page 174)
PLUS
APPLE AND BLACKCURRANT WHIP
(see recipe, page 173)

WARM UP – MOBILITY AND PULSE-RAISING

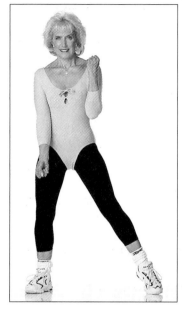

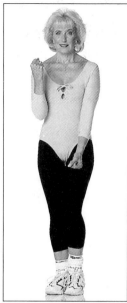

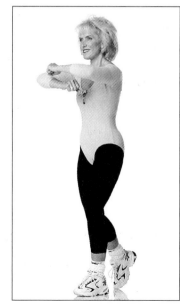

▲ **1 Step Touch with Bicep Curls** Stand tall and step out to alternate sides, bending your knees as the feet come together. At the same time bend alternate elbows, keeping them close to the waist. Perform 16 times altogether.

2 Walks with Arm Rolls Walk forward for 3 counts, rolling the arms at chest height, and on the 4th count bring the feet together and clap, then walk backwards again and clap. Stand tall, with your head up and your tummy pulled in. Move forward and back 4 times altogether.

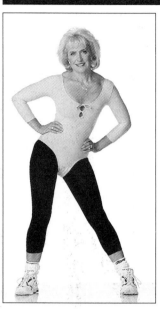

4 Hopscotch with Elbow Presses
Take a step out to the side on the right leg and bend the left leg up behind. At the same time have your elbows up at shoulder height and, as the leg lifts at the back, press the elbows behind you, then repeat to the other side. Now make the steps wider and use the arms more strongly to make the move more effective. Repeat 16 times altogether.

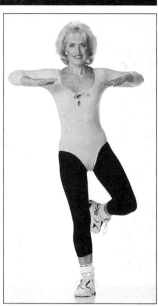

6 Calf Stretch
Stand upright, with one foot in front of the other. Keep the back leg straight and bend the front leg and make sure both feet point forward. Lean towards the front leg to feel a stretch in the lower leg at the back. Now take the back leg further back to gain a more effective stretch. Hold for 8 seconds, then change legs and repeat.

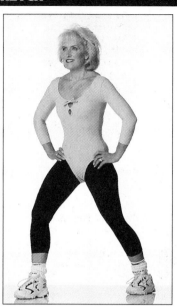

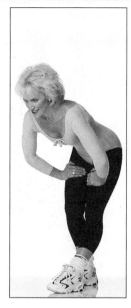

▲ **3 Hip Rolls** With feet wide apart and knees bent, roll the hips around in a full circle, from the side, round to the front, and then to the back. Keep it very smooth and under control. Repeat 4 times slowly in one direction and then change direction.

5 Squats with Arms With feet apart, bend from the knees, letting your hips dip back as if you were trying to sit in a chair. At the same time, draw your arms straight up in front of you to shoulder height. Look straight ahead, keeping your back flat and your tummy pulled in tight against your spine. Do 8 altogether.

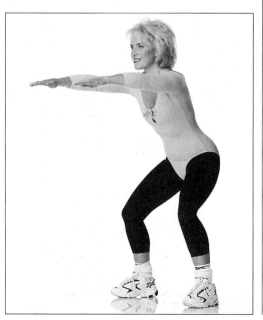

8 Front of Thigh Stretch Stand up straight and take hold around one ankle so that the knee points towards the floor and the knees are fairly close together. Try to keep the knee of the supporting leg slightly bent and push the hip forward on the held leg to feel the stretch down the front of the thigh. Hold for 8 seconds, then change legs and repeat.

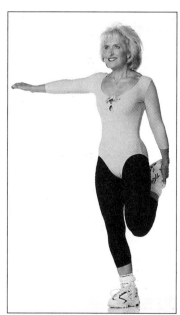

▲ **7 Back of Thigh Stretch** Stand with your back leg bent and your front leg straight, and place your hands in the middle of your thighs. Now, keeping your head up and your back flat, lean forward until you feel a stretch in the back of the straight leg. Hold for 8 seconds, then change legs and repeat.

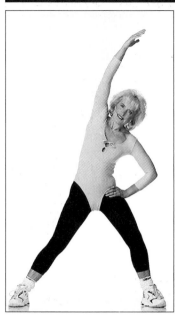

9 Inner Thigh and Waist Stretch
Stand with feet wide apart, and start with an inner thigh stretch by bending your right knee in line with the toes and keeping the left leg straight, with the foot pointing forward. Feel the stretch in the inner thigh. Now take your left arm up over your head and lean slightly to the right to feel the stretch in your waist. Hold for 8 seconds, then repeat to the other side.

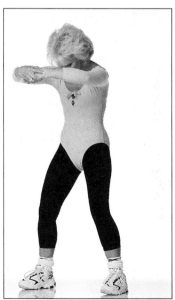

10 Upper Back Stretch Standing with feet comfortably apart, bring your arms round in front of your chest and clasp your hands together. Drop your head forward and gently press the arms away from the hands to feel a stretch across the shoulder blades at the back. Hold for 6 seconds, then release.

SEQUENCE 1

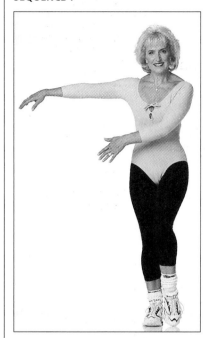

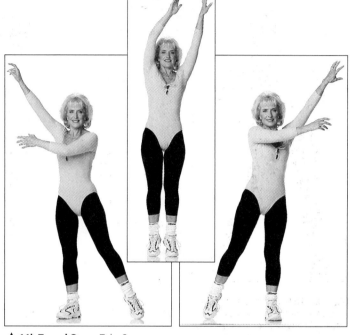

11a Step Touch Swing Step from side to side, swinging your arms above shoulder height. Keep the move controlled and keep your head up and your shoulders well back, but try to work really hard with each step. Do 8 before changing to 11b.

▲ 11b Travel Overs Take 2 steps to the side, swinging your arms over in the direction you are moving. Add a little jump as the feet come together, making sure both heels land on the floor each time. Repeat twice to each side before moving on to 11c.

11c Touch Backs As you come back from the final travel over, take your right leg back to touch the toe to the floor behind you. As you change to the other leg take a small spring between each touch back so that you work harder. Do 8 before moving on to Sequence 2.

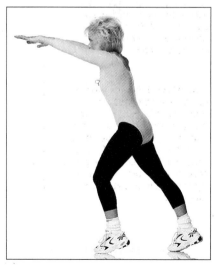

SEQUENCE 2

12a Hopscotch with High Arms Take a step out to the side on the right leg, taking your arms high above your head. Now, as you bend the left leg up behind draw the arms strongly down by your sides to finish the move. Change to the other side and keep alternating sides for 8 repetitions before moving on to 12b.

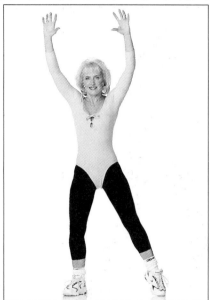

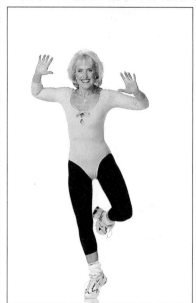

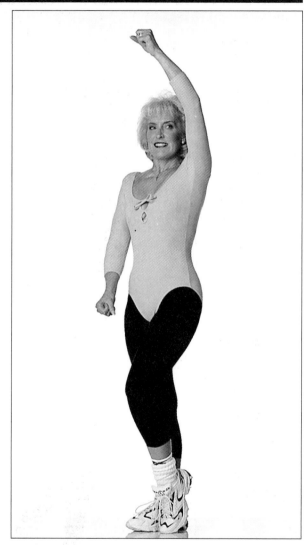

12b Walks with Rolling Arms Take 3 steps forward, then bring the feet together with a jump and a clap on the 4th count. Repeat moving backwards. Roll the arms at chest height as you travel and aim to cover more ground and take bigger jumps as the routine progresses. Repeat forward and back twice before moving on to 12c.

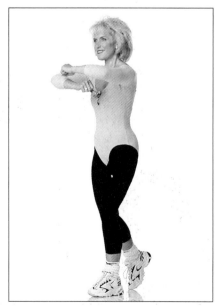

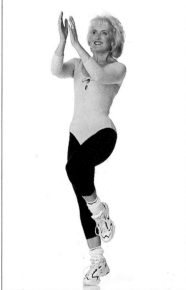

12c Skip Turns with Punching Arms Take 4 full counts to turn all the way round with a jumping skip, really lifting the knees now, and punch alternate arms up in the air as you skip. Then go back the other way. Check the heels land on the floor each time you skip, control the arm movement and keep tall. Now move on to Sequence 3.

SEQUENCE 3

13a Box Step with High Arms Take a step forward with the right leg, leading with the heel, with the right arm overhead. Now do the same on the left side. As you step back with alternate legs, draw your elbows behind you at waist height with 2 little pushes. Step wide and use the arms strongly but keep your body upright. Do 4 box steps before moving on to 13b.

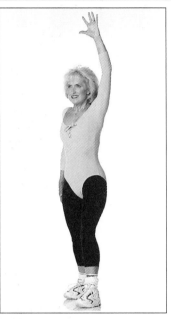
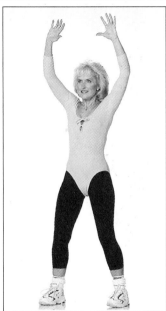
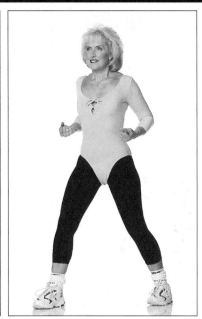

13b Half Jacks with Arms Take alternate toes out to the sides, bringing your arms out to just above shoulder height at the same time. As you change from one foot to the other add a small spring to increase the intensity of the move. Repeat 8 times under control before moving on to 13c.

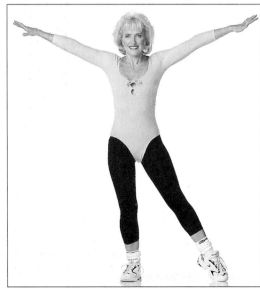

13c Double Scoops with Claps On the last half jack, turn to your right and make a scooping action with both arms as you lead off with the heel of the right foot, bringing the left foot up close behind. Take another scoop to the right, adding a clap and a jump before turning to go left. Repeat a double scoop to each side before moving on to Sequence 4.

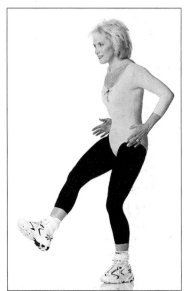
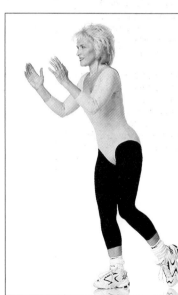

SEQUENCE 4

14a Grapevine with Arm Circles
Take a grapevine to your right and as the feet come together at the end take 2 knee bends with a little jump off the floor, circling the arms in front of you at the same time. Now take a grapevine back to the left with 2 knee bends and arm circles on the end. Repeat twice through before moving on to 14b.

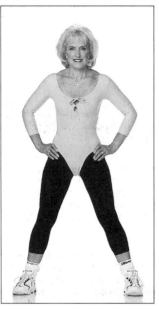
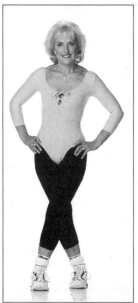
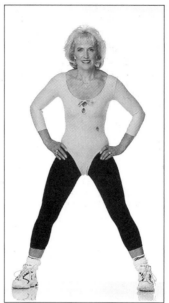
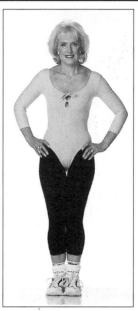
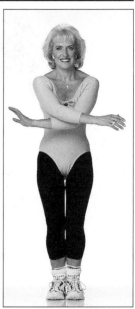

14b Alternate Squats with Jumps Next take a large squat step out to the right, really bending your knees and taking your hips back. As you come up again bring the feet together and do 2 small jumps with claps. Now do exactly the same out to the left. Keep your head up and your back straight all the time. Repeat 4 times altogether before moving on to 14c.

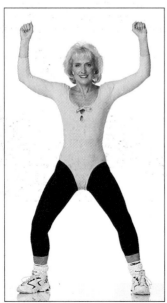
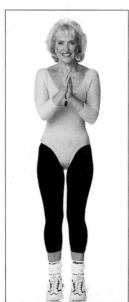
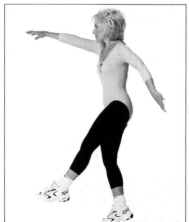
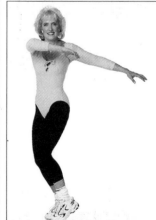

14c Kick Away Forward and Twist Back Take a step forward on the right foot and continue to travel forward as you kick the left leg forward. Keep alternating legs, travelling forward until you have completed 4 kicks. Now twist backwards for 4 counts. Stand tall throughout and make sure those heels go down as you land. Repeat twice through before going back to Sequence 1.

Keep repeating the sequences until you feel you have worked long and hard enough to suit your ability.

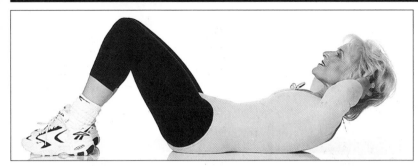

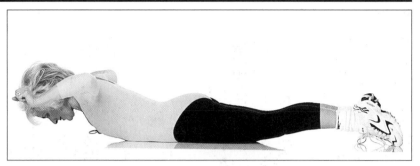

15 Abdominal Curl Lie on your back, with your knees bent and your feet flat on the floor. Place your hands at the sides of your head to support your neck. Now pull your tummy in towards your spine and hold it in as you lift just the head and shoulders off the floor, then lower them again. Breathe out as you lift, and breathe in as you lower. Repeat 8 times slowly, then rest and repeat.

16 Posture Improver and Spine Strengthener Lie on your front, with both arms out to the sides in line with your shoulders, as shown. Now carefully squeeze the shoulders on count 1, then lift the upper body from the floor on count 2. Lower the upper body down to the floor on count 3, then finally lower the shoulders to the floor on count 4 to finish. Keep the movement controlled, breathing out as you lift and breathing in as you lower. Repeat 4 times, then rest and repeat 4 more.

◀ **17 Bottom and Back of Thigh Toner** Come up onto your forearms and knees, with your tummy pulled in tight and your back held flat. Extend your right leg out so that the toe is on the floor. Now lift the leg to hip height, then bend the knee pulling the heel toward the hip, extend the leg again, then lower it to the floor. Repeat 8 times, then change legs and repeat.

18 Inner Thigh Toner Lie on your side and place the top leg over the underneath leg, still using the towel under the knee for extra comfort if you wish. Smoothly lift the underneath leg, then lower it again. Repeat 16 times, then rest and repeat. Roll over and repeat with the other leg.

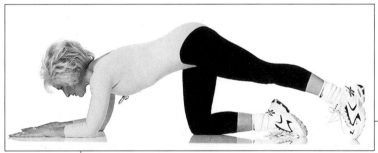

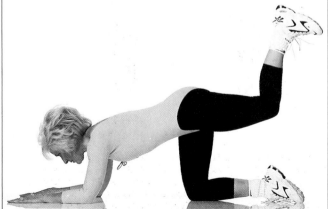

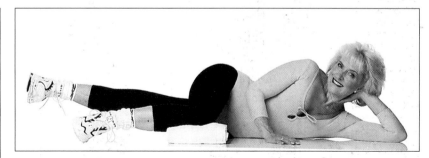

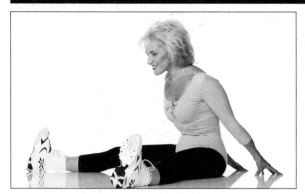

19 Inner Thigh Stretch Sit with your legs comfortably wide apart, and lift up tall, with your back straight and your head up. Place your hands behind your hips and use them to help you push your pelvis further forward. Now lean forward, still keeping your back straight, and feel a strong stretch in the inner thighs. Hold for 10 seconds, then take a deep breath in and, as you breathe out, lean further forward to hold for another 10 seconds.

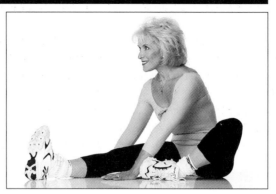

20 Back of Thigh Stretch Sit up, with one leg diagonally out in front of you and the other leg tucked up in front of the hip as shown. Place your hands to either side of the straight leg and, keeping your back flat and your head up, lean forward slightly to feel a stretch in the back of the thigh. Hold for 10 seconds, then try to lean even further forward, without bending the spine, to develop the stretch more, and hold for a further 10 seconds. Change legs and repeat.

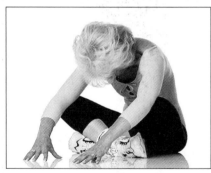

21 Spine Stretch Sit with legs comfortably crossed and place your hands in front of you on the floor. Lower your head and slide the hands further along the floor to feel a stretch along your spine. Hold for 8 seconds, then release.

▶ **23 Front of Thigh Stretch** Lying on your front, bend your right knee up and take hold of the ankle. Ease the heel close to the hip and push that hip firmly into the floor. Hold for 10 seconds, then change legs and repeat.

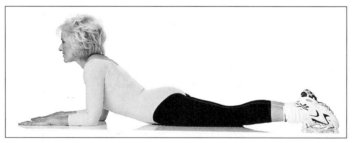

22 Abdominal Stretch Lie on your front, place your bent arms in front of you and prop yourself up on your elbows, keeping the whole of each forearm on the floor. Now gently lift the chin forward slightly to feel a stretch down the front of the trunk. Hold for 6 seconds, then rest.

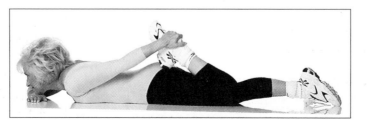

POSITIVE THOUGHT FOR THE DAY

On Day 16 we started making plans for our tangible and intangible goals. I hope you have written some of them down and also started thinking very creatively about achieving some of the short-term ones as well as making long-term plans for the more ambitious ones. It is important to write these plans down and to keep them under review. If we go on holiday, we are meticulous in our arrangements – checking our passport, planning our wardrobe, organising injections, traveller's cheques and currency. We often make a careful list which we check off as we do each job. It is not only easier to remember everything this way, but it can actually be more fun too. There is a real sense of achievement when everything has been ticked off and we can rest easy knowing that everything is under control. However, we didn't write that list at one go. We would have started with the priorities and gradually added items as they occurred to us. In other words, the subconscious was working in an expanding way, trying to think of anything that might have been overlooked. Lying in bed at night is a perfect time for scanning our brain for those things we might have forgotten. I always keep a notepad by my bedside to record such thoughts and, this way, I can be confident that I really have thought of everything.

We exercise such good sense and creative effort when going on holiday, but we hardly plan our lives at all! If we took half the amount of effort in planning for the future, we would be much more certain of making that a success too.

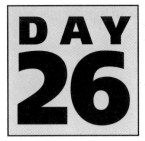

DAY 26

Today I would like you to consider your attitude towards work. Wouldn't it be great if you didn't consider your job to be actual work because you really enjoyed it?

I can honestly say I hardly do any of what I would call 'work', even though I am involved in various projects that occupy me through my working week. But, because I really enjoy it all, how can I call it work? Am I just lucky? No, definitely not. My life is organised in such a way that I have excluded the jobs I like least. Removing the 'job weeds' from my life has made for a less stressful lifestyle and I actually look forward to every day.

We are all in control of our future and our happiness. It doesn't just happen. Consider today whether you look upon your job as 'work' or as an enjoyable way to earn a living.

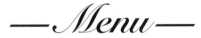

— Menu —

BREAKFAST
1 small bread roll (25g/1oz) spread with a little mustard and filled with 50g (2oz) smoked turkey breast and 2 sliced tomatoes

OR

225g (8oz) tinned grapefruit in natural juice topped with 1 × 150g (5oz) diet yogurt, any flavour

LUNCH
75g (3oz) smoked mackerel or cottage cheese served with CARROT SALAD (see recipe, page 175), COLESLAW (see recipe, page 176), lettuce, tomatoes and cucumber, plus 115g (4oz) grapes

DINNER
115g (4oz) gammon steak (all fat removed) served with 1 slice of pineapple, 115g (4oz) potatoes, unlimited other vegetables and PINEAPPLE SAUCE (see recipe, page 180)

PLUS

RASPBERRY FLUFF
(see recipe, page 181)

OR

VEGETABLE RISOTTO
(see recipe, page 184)

PLUS

RASPBERRY AND STRAWBERRY BAVAROIS
(see recipe, page 181)

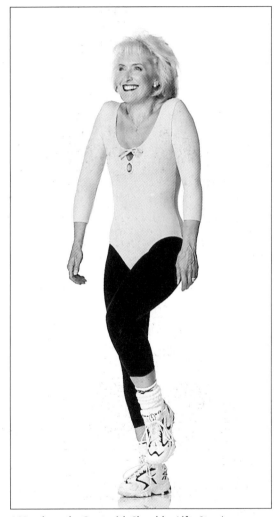

1 March on the Spot with Shoulder Lifts Stand up straight, with your head up and your shoulders back, and march on the spot. As you march, lift both shoulders up towards your ears and then down again, keeping the action slow and controlled. Lift the shoulders for 2 marches and then lower them for 2 to keep a rhythmical pace. Lift and lower the shoulders 8 times altogether.

2 Side Bends with Twists
2a Standing with feet apart, shoulders back and head up, lean slightly to the right, reaching your right arm out and lifting the left elbow up. Come up and lean to the other side. Do 4 repetitions, then change to 2b.

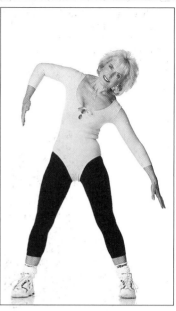

2b Bring the arms up in line with the shoulders as shown and, keeping your hips facing forward, twist the upper body round to the right. Come back to face front and repeat to the left. Do 4 repetitions and then repeat 2a and 2b once more.

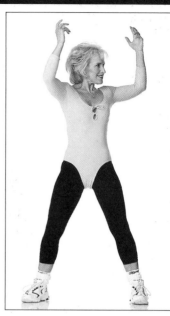

3 Hopscotch with Elbow Presses
Take a step out to the side on the right leg and bend the left leg up behind. At the same time have your elbows up at shoulder height and, as the leg lifts at the back, press the elbows behind you, then repeat to the other side. Now make the steps wider and use the arms more strongly to make the move more effective. Repeat 16 times altogether.

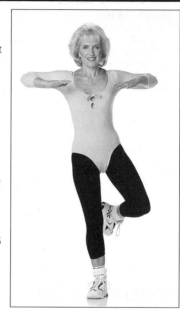

4 Twisted Heel/Toe Take the right heel diagonally out in front on the floor. Keep it there as you twist from the hip and change to the toe. Alternate from heel to toe to a count of 8 then repeat to the left side.

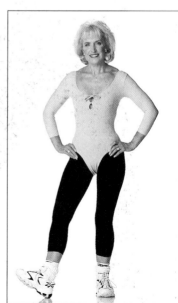

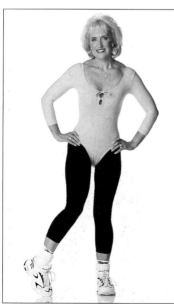

5 Half Jacks with Arms Stand in a good posture and take the right foot out to the side, touching the floor with just the toe. At the same time lift both arms to just above shoulder height. Bring the feet together and repeat to the other side. Repeat 16 times.

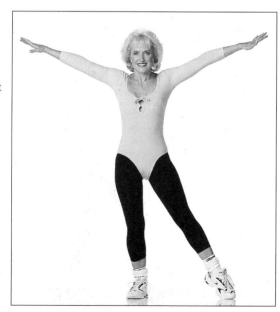

6 Tricep Stretch
Stand with feet apart, tummy pulled in tight and knees slightly bent. Take your right hand behind the right shoulder and use the left hand on the fleshy part of the right underarm to push it further back. Keep your head up throughout and hold for 8 seconds. Change arms and repeat.

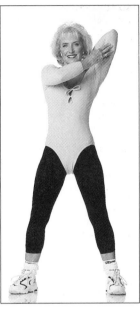

7 Inner Thigh and Waist Stretch
Stand with feet wide apart, and start with an inner thigh stretch by bending your right knee in line with the toes and keeping the left leg straight, with the foot pointing forward. Feel the stretch in the inner thigh. Now take your left arm up over your head and lean slightly to the right to feel the stretch in your waist. Hold for 8 seconds, then repeat to the other side.

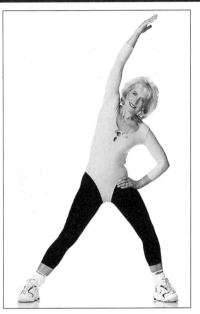

8 Calf Stretch Stand upright, with one foot in front of the other. Keep the back leg straight and bend the front leg and make sure both feet point forward. Lean towards the front leg to feel a stretch in the lower leg at the back. Now take the back leg further back to gain a more effective stretch. Hold for 8 seconds, then change legs and repeat.

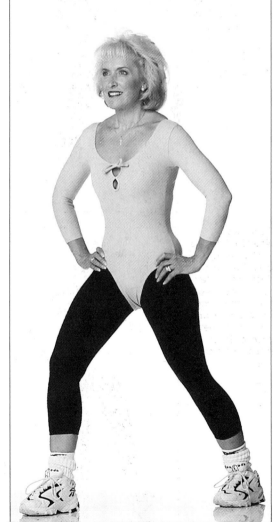

9 Lower Calf and Chest Stretch Place your right leg slightly behind the left leg and bend both knees. Keep both heels firmly on the floor and keep the hips tucked under to feel a stretch further down the calf on the right leg. Now take both hands and either clasp them behind you or place them in the small of your back and squeeze your shoulders back to feel a stretch across your chest. Keep your head up and your back straight at all times. Hold for 8 seconds, then release.

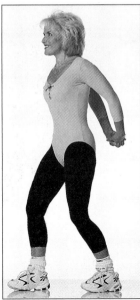

10 Lower Calf and Upper Back Stretch Place the left leg slightly behind the right leg and bend both knees. Keep both heels firmly on the floor and keep the hips tucked under to feel a stretch in the lower left leg. Now bring both arms round in front at chest height, drop your head forward and press your arms away from your upper back to feel a stretch in the upper back. Hold for 8 seconds, then release.

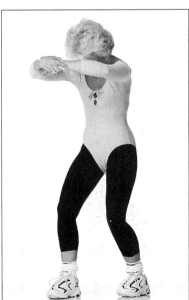

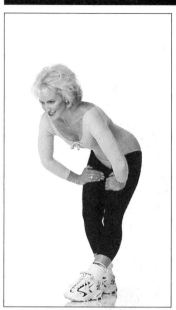

11 Back of Thigh Stretch Stand with your back leg bent and your front leg straight, and place your hands in the middle of your thighs. Now, keeping your head up and your back flat, lean forward until you feel a stretch in the back of the straight leg. Hold for 8 seconds, then change legs and repeat.

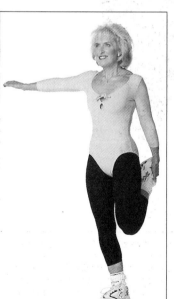

12 Front of Thigh Stretch Stand up straight and take hold around one ankle so that the knee points towards the floor and the knees are fairly close together. Try to keep the knee of the supporting leg slightly bent and push the hip forward on the held leg to feel the stretch down the front of the thigh. Hold for 8 seconds, then change legs and repeat.

SEQUENCE 1

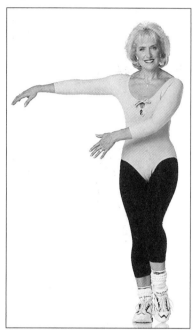

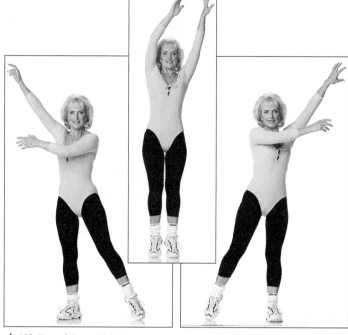

13a Step Touch Swing Step from side to side, swinging your arms above shoulder height. Keep the move controlled, with your head up and your shoulders well back, but try to work really hard with each step. Do 8 before changing to 13b.

▲ **13b Travel Overs** Take 2 steps to the side, swinging your arms over in the direction you are moving. Add a little jump as the feet come together, making sure both heels land on the floor each time. Repeat twice to each side before moving on to 13c.

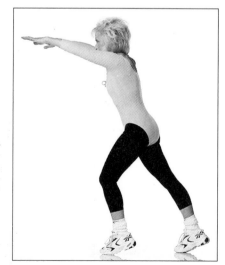

13c Touch Backs As you come back from the final travel over, take your right leg back to touch the toe to the floor behind you. As you change to the other leg take a small spring between each touch back so that you work harder. Do 8 before moving on to Sequence 2.

SEQUENCE 2

14a Hopscotch with High Arms Take a step out to the side on the right leg, taking your arms high above your head. Now, as you bend the left leg up behind draw the arms strongly down by your sides to finish the move. Change to the other side and keep alternating sides for 8 repetitions before moving on to 14b.

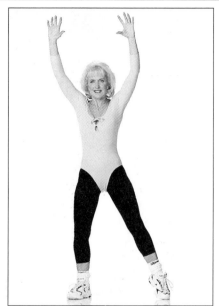

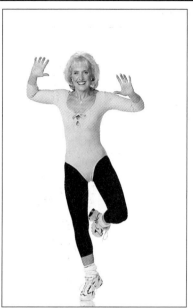

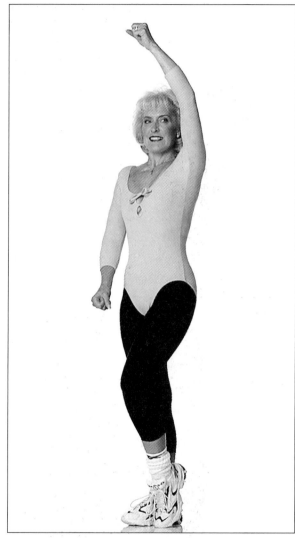

14b Walks with Rolling Arms Take 3 steps forward, then bring the feet together with a jump and a clap on the 4th count. Repeat moving backwards. Roll the arms at chest height as you travel and aim to cover more ground and take bigger jumps as the routine progresses. Repeat forward and back twice before moving on to 14c.

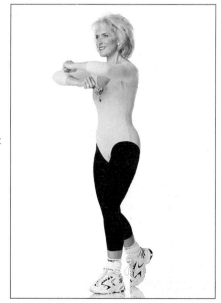

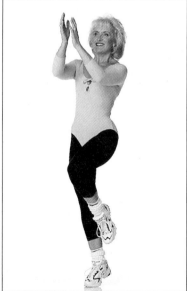

14c Skip Turns with Punching Arms Take 4 full counts to turn all the way round with a jumping skip, really lifting the knees now, and punch alternate arms up in the air as you skip. Then go back the other way. Check the heels land on the floor each time you skip, control the arm movement and keep tall. Now move on to Sequence 3.

SEQUENCE 3

15a Box Step with High Arms Take a step forward with the right leg, leading with the heel, with the right arm overhead. Now do the same on the left side. As you step back with alternate legs, draw your elbows behind you at waist height with 2 little pushes. Step wide and use the arms strongly but keep your body upright. Do 4 box steps before moving on to 15b.

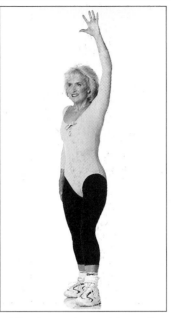
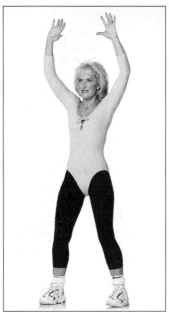
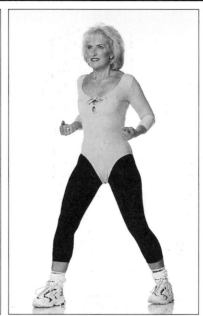

15b Half Jacks with Arms Take alternate toes out to the sides, bringing your arms out to just above shoulder height at the same time. As you change from one foot to the other add a small spring to increase the intensity of the move. Repeat 8 times under control before moving on to 15c.

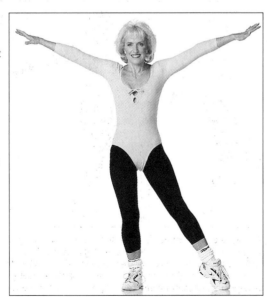

15c Double Scoops with Claps On the last half jack, turn to your right and make a scooping action with both arms as you lead off with the heel of the right foot, bringing the left foot up close behind. Take another scoop to the right, adding a clap and a jump before turning to go left. Repeat a double scoop to each side before moving on to Sequence 4.

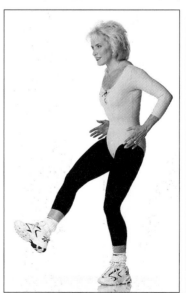
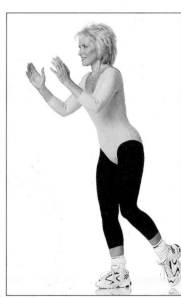

SEQUENCE 4

16a Grapevine with Arm Circles

Take a grapevine to your right and as the feet come together at the end take 2 knee bends with a little jump off the floor, circling the arms in front of you at the same time. Now take a grapevine back to the left with 2 knee bends and arm circles on the end. Repeat twice through before moving on to 16b.

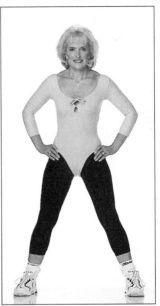 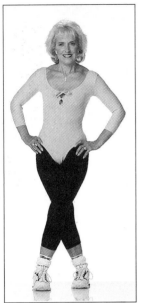 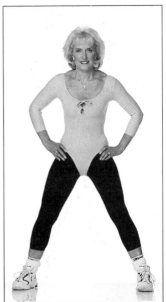 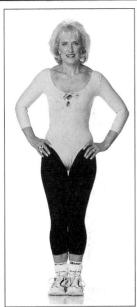 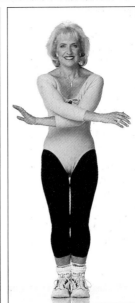

16b Alternate Squats with Jumps

Next take a large squat step out to the right, really bending your knees and taking your hips back. As you come up again bring the feet together and do 2 small jumps with claps. Now do exactly the same out to the left. Keep your head up and your back straight all the time. Repeat 4 times altogether before moving on to 16c.

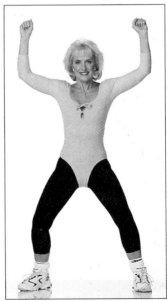 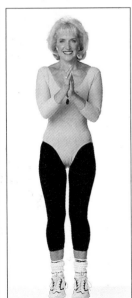 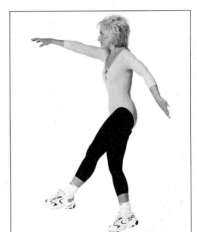 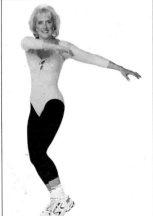

16c Kick Away Forward and Twist Back

Take a step forward on the right foot and continue to travel forward as you kick the left leg forward. Keep alternating legs, travelling forward until you have completed 4 kicks. Now twist backwards for 4 counts. Stand tall throughout and make sure those heels go down as you land. Repeat twice through before going back to Sequence 1.

Keep repeating the sequences until you have completed your full 15 minutes.

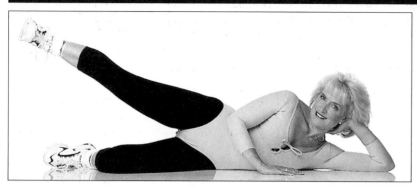

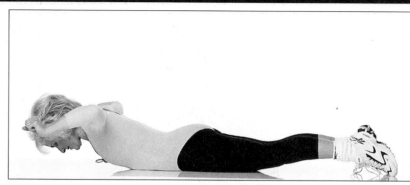

17 Outer Thigh Toner Lie on your side, with your head propped on your elbow. Bend the bottom leg and keep the top leg in a straight line from your shoulder. Now lift the top leg halfway through the range, then hold momentarily before continuing to lift to just above hip height. On the way down, pause again at the halfway mark and hold momentarily before lowering the leg to the floor. Perform 12 times slowly and under control, then roll over and repeat on the other leg.

19 Posture Improver and Spine Strengthener Lie on your front, with both arms out to the sides in line with your shoulders. Now carefully squeeze the shoulders on count 1, then lift the upper body from the floor on count 2. Lower the upper body down to the floor on count 3, then finally lower the shoulders to the floor on count 4 to finish. Keep the movement controlled, breathing out as you lift and breathing in as you lower. Repeat 4 times, then rest and repeat 4 more.

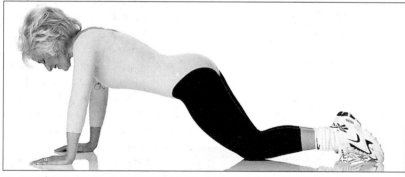

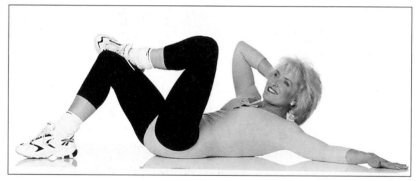

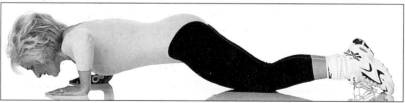

18 Elongated Press Ups Come up onto your hands and knees and pull your tummy in tight to flatten your back. Make sure your hands are directly underneath your shoulders but now take the knee further back as shown, to increase the weight carried by the arms. Now lower and lift the upper body, taking care not to lock the elbows out at the top. Breathe out as you lift and breathe in as you lower. Do 6 repetitions, then rest and repeat.

20 Waist Crunches Lie on your back, with your right leg bent and the foot flat on the floor. Now place your left ankle across the knee of the right leg, allowing the left knee to drop outwards slightly. Place your right hand behind your head for support and place your left arm out straight, at a right angle to the body. Now pull your tummy in against your spine and lift your upper body, bringing your right shoulder towards your left knee. Breathe out as you lift and in as you lower. Lift 8 times, then change sides and repeat.

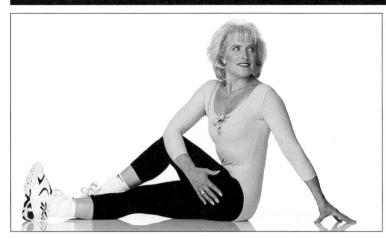

21 Outer Thigh and Waist Stretch Sit upright, with both legs out in front. Take your right leg across the left leg and place the right foot in line with the left knee. Now place your left arm over the right knee to squeeze it further across the chest to feel a stretch in the outer thigh. Now twist your trunk around to the right to feel a stretch in your waist. Try to keep your back lifted and your head up at all times. Hold for 8 seconds, then change sides and repeat.

23 Tricep Stretch Sitting with legs crossed, head up and shoulders back, place your right hand behind your right shoulder and take the left hand across in front to push the arm further back. Hold for 6 seconds, then change sides and repeat.

22 Chest Stretch Sit with your legs crossed, your back straight and your head up. Take both hands behind you and clasp them loosely. Now keeping your elbows bent, squeeze your shoulders back to feel a stretch across your chest. Hold for 8 seconds, then release.

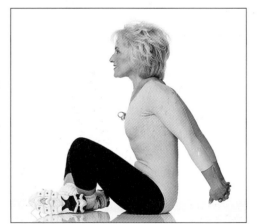

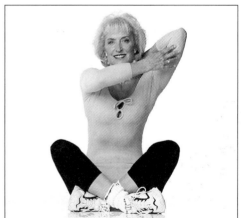

24 Front of Thigh Stretch Lie on your front, bend your right knee up and take hold of the ankle. Ease the heel close to the hip and push that hip firmly into the floor. Hold for 10 seconds, then change legs and repeat.

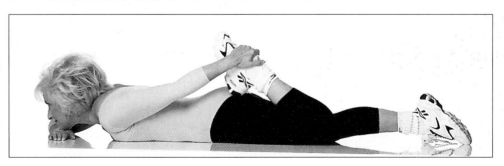

POSITIVE THOUGHT FOR THE DAY

In these last days of the programme I am asking you to work your body harder. It is a wonderful feeling to be able to experience the increased fitness and strength that you have built up over the last few weeks. I am sure you will be feeling that it has been worthwhile.

Just as you have challenged your body beyond what you had previously thought possible, so you can extend your mind. The times we hear ourselves saying, 'I'd really love to have a go at such and such a thing, but I know I couldn't do it.' How do you know? Even if you have tried once and failed, what is to stop you having another go? Often when ladies come along to join my class, they say: 'I can't get below 10st (63.5kg).' Why? Because, up to this point, they haven't achieved a lower weight and they have conditioned themselves into believing they can't. While they believe that, they won't! We must break down the barriers of conditioning and open our minds to far higher goals.

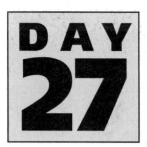

The last but one day of this programme and I hope you are feeling good. Take a rest from the formal exercises today, but remember you are going to have to work extra hard tomorrow so that you achieve optimum benefits for your figure before you take that 'after' photograph.

Start planning your celebration for the day of the last measuring session – the day after tomorrow.

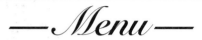

BREAKFAST

25g (1oz) very lean bacon or 2 turkey rashers, grilled and served on
25g (1oz) toast with 2 grilled tomatoes

OR

225g (8oz) fruit compote (mixed tinned fruit in natural juice) topped with
75g (3oz) diet yogurt

LUNCH

Jacket potato (approx. 175g/6oz) topped with COLESLAW (see recipe, page 176),
plus 1 × 150g (5oz) diet yogurt

OR

175g (6oz) low-fat cottage cheese served with large mixed salad in OIL-FREE
ORANGE AND LEMON VINAIGRETTE DRESSING (see recipe, page 179),
plus 115g (4oz) grapes

DINNER

Any ready meal with a maximum of 300kcals and 4% fat. Serve with
unlimited vegetables
PLUS
STRAWBERRY WINE JELLY (see recipe, page 183)

OR

Any ready vegetarian meal with a maximum of 300kcals and 4% fat.
Serve with unlimited vegetables
PLUS
COEURS A LA CREME (see recipe, page 176)

POSITIVE THOUGHT FOR THE DAY

Smiling and laughing is a terrific tonic for everyone. Now that you've reached the end of Day 27, you have every reason to smile. Not only have you achieved a real goal – well, almost – but from now on there will be no more excuses, no more 'false ceilings' for projects and ambitions. This is just the beginning of a very new and different life for you.

Do you feel ambitious enough to attain goals that previously you might have thought were out of your personal reach? Success is not about money or position, it is about personal satisfaction and self-esteem. We must have confidence in ourselves; if we don't, how can we expect someone else to? The only way to build self-confidence is to keep on having a go at goal-scoring. Everyone is inspired by a successful person. They want to be part of the action too. And, amazing though it might seem, you will attract new friends who want to be like you. So next time someone copies what you are wearing, or wants to know how you got into shape, take it as a real compliment.

DAY 28

Can you believe it – this is the last day of the New Inch Loss Plan? Tomorrow is the final weighing and measuring session for this 28-day period. I hope you will be particularly strong today so that tomorrow you can achieve the best possible results. Exercise with energy, diet with even greater dedication and look forward to the future with total determination.

I hope at this point your self-image has improved dramatically. I am only too well aware that few are fortunate enough to have a perfect body – very few in fact. That aside, we should all try to be happy with the body we have. This 28-day programme should have given you the opportunity to come to terms with your body. I am still very critical of my own shape, but I console myself with the fact that, while it is far from perfect, it is better than it used to be. If I stopped exercising and simply ate everything I wanted, I know it would be a very different shape. It is worth the effort because I feel so much better about it now than I did before discovering the benefits of low-fat eating and regular exercise. I'm not ashamed of my body any more. That's the difference it has made to me. I hope it will do the same for you too. Enjoy this last day and get ready for that celebration tomorrow. Make sure you have a film in your camera and be prepared to have your 'after' photograph taken in the morning.

—Menu—

BREAKFAST

2 bananas mashed with 15g (1/2oz) chopped sultanas and topped with 75g (3oz) diet yogurt

OR

1 whole fresh grapefruit, 1 slice of wholemeal bread and 2 teaspoons of marmalade

LUNCH

175g (6oz) fresh salmon steak served with 115g (4oz) new potatoes and unlimited vegetables such as mangetout, asparagus or broccoli and served with PARSLEY SAUCE (see recipe, page 179)
PLUS
CHOCOLATE AND COFFEE ROULADE (see recipe, page 175)

OR

LENTIL ROAST (see recipe, page 178)
PLUS
APRICOT PLUM SOFTIE (see recipe, page 173)

SUPPER

75g (3oz) wafer thin chicken served with large salad including CARROT SALAD (see recipe, page 175) and OIL-FREE ORANGE AND LEMON VINAIGRETTE DRESSING (see recipe, page 179), plus 115g (4oz) fresh fruit salad served in a meringue basket

OR

Jacket potato (approx. 175g/6oz) topped with 115g (4oz) low-fat cottage cheese and served with a large salad including beansprouts, grated carrots, grated raw beetroot and soy sauce, plus 75g (3oz) low-fat fromage frais

WARM UP – MOBILITY AND PULSE-RAISING

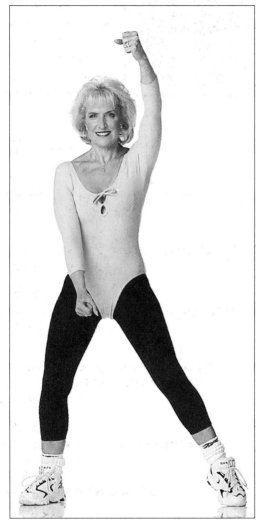

1 Side Steps with Monkey Arms Take 2 steps out to the right, with your arms straight out in front, pulling them up and down alternately in rhythm with the steps. Take 2 steps back to the left and keep going, to repeat the sequence 4 times altogether.

2 Squats with Figure of 8 Arms

Stand with feet apart and take a rhythmical squat, making sure the knees bend in the direction of the toes. At the same time make a figure of 8 with your arms in front of you. Do 16 altogether.

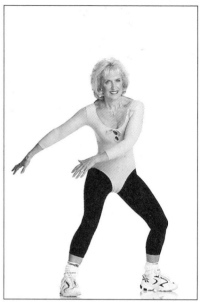

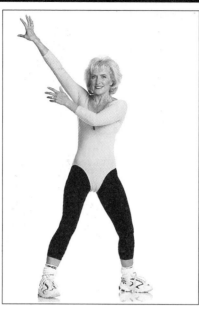

3 Weight Transfer with Arm Circles

Transfer your weight from one foot to the other and at the same time take the opposite arm in a circling action just above the head. So, as you take the weight to the right leg, the left arm goes over and so on. Control the move and pull your tummy in and maintain a good posture. Repeat 16 times altogether.

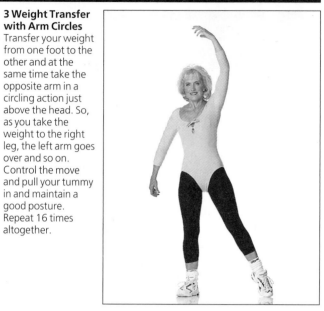

4 Touch Backs with Arms

Start with feet together, then take one foot behind you, touching the floor with just the toe. At the same time reach both arms forward to chest height. You can lean forward slightly but make sure your tummy is in tight to support your back. Keep changing legs and repeat 12 times altogether.

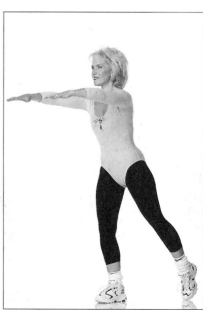

5 Heel/Toe with Bicep Curls

Take the right heel out diagonally in front on the floor and then change to the toe. At the same time bend alternate elbows, keeping them close to the waist and under control. Rhythmically keep changing from heel to toe for 4 counts, counting 1 every time the heel strikes the floor. Change legs and repeat, then repeat again on each leg.

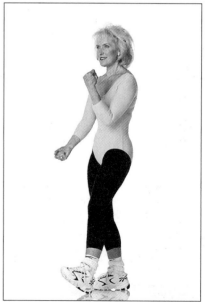

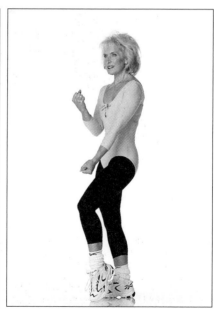

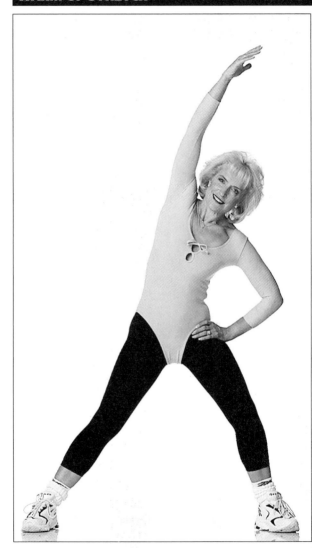

7 Calf Stretch
Stand upright, with one foot in front of the other. Keep the back leg straight and bend the front leg and make sure both feet point forward. Lean towards the front leg to feel a stretch in the lower leg at the back. Now take the back leg further back to gain a more effective stretch. Hold for 8 seconds, then change legs and repeat.

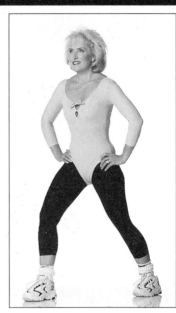

8 Back of Thigh Stretch Stand with your back leg bent and your front leg straight, and place your hands in the middle of your thighs. Now, keeping your head up and your back flat, lean forward until you feel a stretch in the back of the straight leg. Hold for 8 seconds, then change legs and repeat.

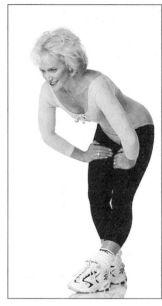

9 Front of Thigh Stretch Stand up straight and take hold around one ankle so that the knee points towards the floor and the knees are fairly close together. Try to keep the knee of the supporting leg slightly bent and push the hip forward on the held leg to feel the stretch down the front of the thigh. Hold for 8 seconds, then change legs and repeat.

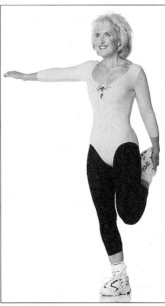
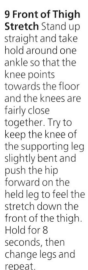

10 Upper Back Stretch Standing with feet comfortably apart, bring your arms round in front of your chest and clasp your hands together. Drop your head forward and gently press the arms away from the hands to feel a stretch across the shoulder blades at the back. Hold for 6 seconds, then release.

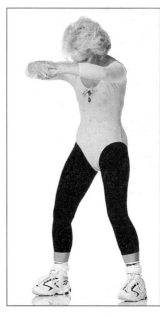

6 Inner Thigh and Waist Stretch Stand with feet wide apart, and start with an inner thigh stretch by bending your right knee in line with the toes and keeping the left leg straight, with the foot pointing forward. Feel the stretch in the inner thigh. Now take your left arm up over your head and lean slightly to the right to feel the stretch in your waist. Hold for 8 seconds, then repeat to the other side.

SEQUENCE 1

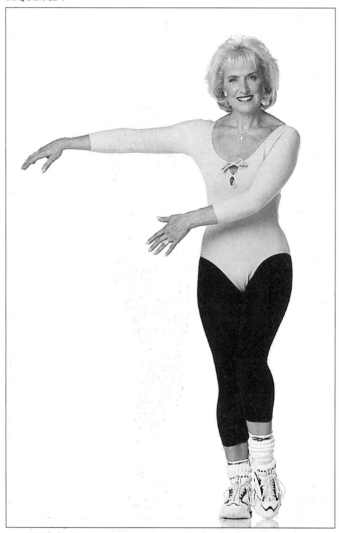

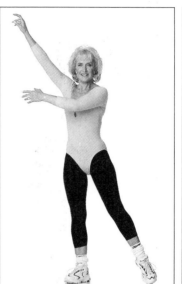 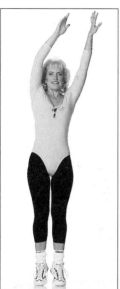 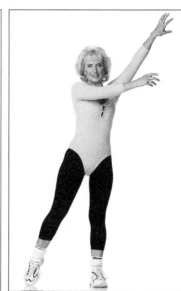

▲ **11b Travel Overs** Take 2 steps to the side, swinging your arms over in the direction you are moving. Add a little jump as the feet come together, making sure both heels land on the floor each time. Repeat twice to each side before moving on to 11c.

11c Touch Backs As you come back from the final travel over, take your right leg back to touch the toe to the floor behind you. As you change to the other leg take a small spring between each touch back so that you work harder. Do 8 before moving on to Sequence 2.

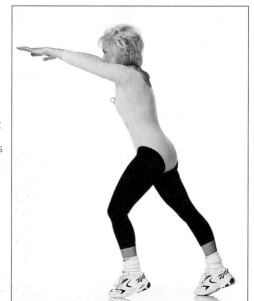

11a Step Touch Swing Step from side to side, swinging your arms above shoulder height. Keep the move controlled, with your head up and your shoulders well back, but try to work really hard with each step. Do 8 before changing to 11b.

SEQUENCE 2

12a Hopscotch with High Arms Take a step out to the side on the right leg, taking your arms high above your head. Now, as you bend the left leg up behind draw the arms strongly down by your sides to finish the move. Change to the other side and keep alternating sides for 8 repetitions before moving on to 12b.

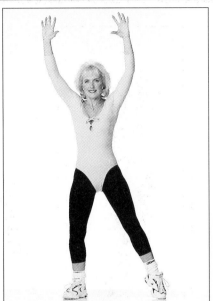

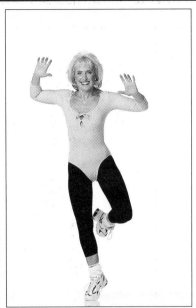

12b Walks with Rolling Arms Take 3 steps forward, then bring the feet together with a jump and a clap on the 4th count. Repeat moving backwards. Roll the arms at chest height as you travel and aim to cover more ground and take bigger jumps as the routine progresses. Repeat forward and back twice before moving on to 12c.

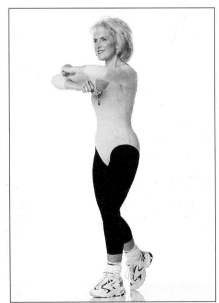

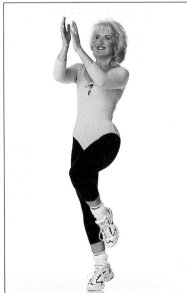

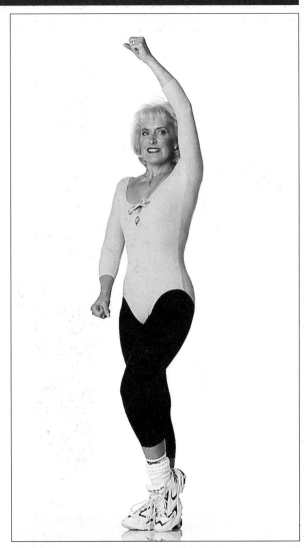

12c Skip Turns with Punching Arms Take 4 full counts to turn all the way round with a jumping skip, really lifting the knees now, and punch alternate arms up in the air as you skip. Then go back the other way. Check the heels land on the floor each time you skip, control the arm movement and keep tall. Now move on to Sequence 3.

SEQUENCE 3

13a Box Step with High Arms Take a step forward with the right leg, leading with the heel, with the right arm overhead. Now do the same on the left side. As you step back with alternate legs, draw your elbows behind you at waist height with 2 little pushes. Step wide and use the arms strongly but keep your body upright. Do 4 box steps before moving on to 13b.

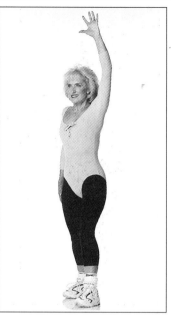
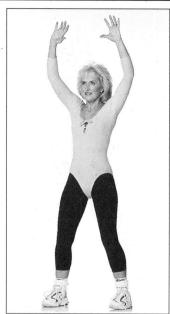
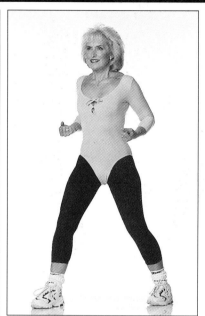

13b Half Jacks with Arms Take alternate toes out to the sides, bringing your arms out to just above shoulder height at the same time. As you change from one foot to the other add a small spring to increase the intensity of the move. Repeat 8 times under control before moving on to 13c.

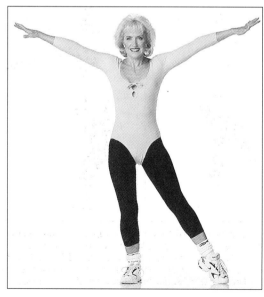

13c Double Scoops with Claps On the last half jack, turn to your right and make a scooping action with both arms as you lead off with the heel of the right foot, bringing the left foot up close behind. Take another scoop to the right, adding a clap and a jump before turning to go left. Repeat a double scoop to each side before moving on to Sequence 4.

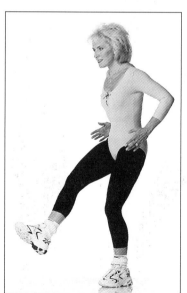
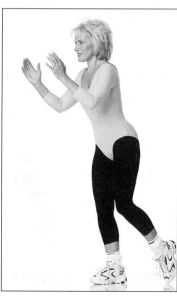

SEQUENCE 4

14a Grapevine with Arm Circles

Take a grapevine to your right and as the feet come together at the end take 2 knee bends with a little jump off the floor, circling the arms in front of you at the same time. Now take a grapevine back to the left with 2 knee bends and arm circles on the end. Repeat twice through before moving on to 14b.

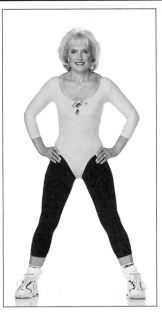
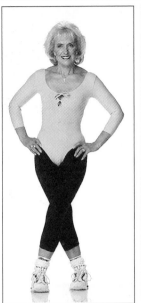
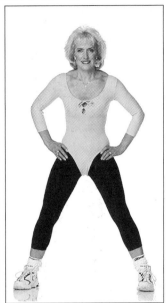
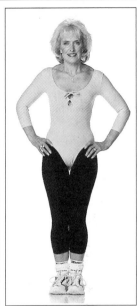
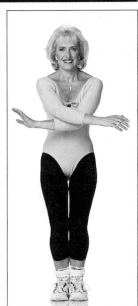

14b Alternate Squats with Jumps

Next take a large squat step out to the right, really bending your knees and taking your hips back. As you come up again bring the feet together and do 2 small jumps with claps. Now do exactly the same out to the left. Keep your head up and your back straight all the time. Repeat 4 times altogether before moving on to 14c.

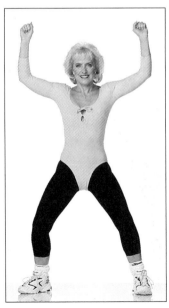
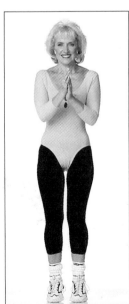
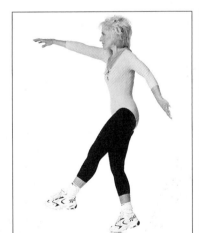
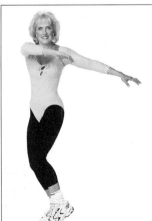

Keep repeating the sequences until you have completed your full 15 minutes.

14c Kick Away Forward and Twist Back

Take a step forward on the right foot and continue to travel forward as you kick the left leg forward. Keep alternating legs, travelling forward until you have completed 4 kicks. Now twist backwards for 4 counts. Stand tall throughout and make sure those heels go down as you land. Repeat twice through before going back to Sequence 1.

15 Abdominal Curl Lie on your back, with your knees bent and your feet flat on the floor. Place your hands at the sides of your head to support your neck. Now pull your tummy in towards your spine and hold it in as you lift just the head and shoulders off the floor, then lower them again. Breathe out as you lift, and breathe in as you lower. Repeat 8 times slowly, then rest and repeat.

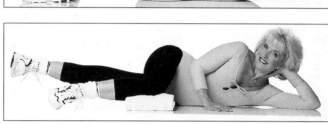

16 Inner Thigh Toner Lie on your side and place the top leg over the underneath leg, still using the towel under the knee for extra comfort if you wish. Smoothly lift the underneath leg, then lower it again. Repeat 16 times, then rest and repeat. Roll over and repeat with the other leg.

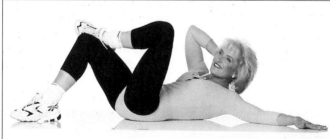

17 Waist Crunches Lie on your back, with your right leg bent and the foot flat on the floor. Now place your left ankle across the knee of the right leg, allowing the left knee to drop outwards slightly. Place your right hand behind your head for support and place your left arm out straight, at a right angle to the body. Now pull your tummy in against your spine and lift your upper body, bringing your right shoulder towards your left knee. Breathe out as you lift, and breathe in as you lower. Lift 8 times, then change sides and repeat.

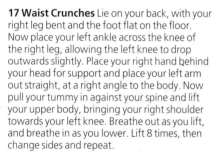

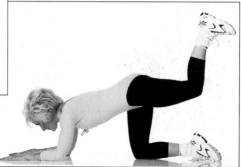

18 Bottom and Back of Thigh Toner Come up onto your forearms and knees, with your tummy pulled in tight and your back held flat. Extend your right leg out so that the toe is on the floor. Now lift the leg to hip height, then bend the knee pulling the heel toward the hip, extend the leg again, then lower it to the floor. Repeat 8 times, then change legs and repeat.

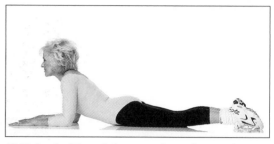

19 Abdominal Stretch Lie on your front, place your bent arms in front of you and prop yourself up on your elbows, keeping the whole of each forearm on the floor. Now gently lift the chin forward slightly to feel a stretch down the front of the trunk. Hold for 6 seconds, then rest.

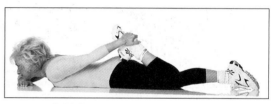

20 Front of Thigh Stretch Lying on your front, bend your right knee up and take hold of the ankle. Ease the heel close to the hip and push that hip firmly into the floor. Hold for 10 seconds, then change legs and repeat.

21 Waist Stretch Sit upright with legs comfortably crossed. Lift your right arm up in the air toward the ceiling and place your left hand on the floor for support. Now, keeping both hips firmly on the floor, lean slightly to the left to feel a stretch down the waist on the right side. Hold for 8 seconds, then release and repeat to the other side.

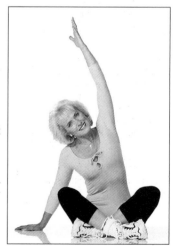

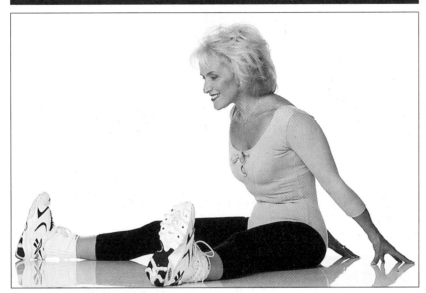

22 Inner Thigh Stretch Sit with your legs comfortably wide apart, and lift up tall, with your back straight and your head up. Place your hands behind your hips and use them to help you push your pelvis further forward. Now lean forward, still keeping your back straight, and feel a strong stretch in the inner thighs. Hold for 10 seconds, then take a deep breath in and, as you breathe out, lean further forward to hold for another 10 seconds.

23 Back of Thigh Stretch Sit up, with one leg diagonally out in front of you and the other leg tucked up in front of the hip as shown. Place your hands to either side of the straight leg and, keeping your back flat and your head up, lean forward slightly to feel a stretch in the back of the thigh. Hold for 10 seconds, then try to lean even further forward, without bending the spine, to develop the stretch more, and hold for a further 10 seconds. Change legs and repeat.

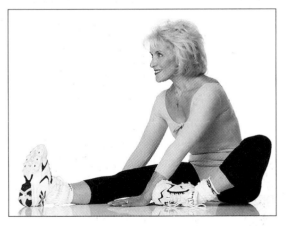

POSITIVE THOUGHT FOR THE DAY

On this last day I want to sum up the things we have discussed. Please use this as a reminder to ensure that you keep up the good work and the resolutions you have started.

1 Your body is now so much improved that you actually feel happier with it.
2 If you are to build self-confidence, you must score lots of goals, no matter how minor these might be.
3 Review your goal plan regularly.
4 Eliminate any previous conditioning that has prevented you from winning in the past.
5 Remember that if you want something badly enough, persistence will win the day.
6 Believe in yourself and do not be sensitive to remarks made by others who want to hurt you. You must try to respond to a negative with a positive.
7 Having a positive attitude makes life so much better.
8 You should try to be happy in everything you do. Try to remove all the 'weeds' from your life.
9 If you are to achieve major goals in your life, you must plan accordingly.
10 Just as you need encouragement from others, so they need it from you. Try to develop the habit of complimenting and encouraging others.
11 When something doesn't go as you had hoped, you must try to see the good that comes out of it in the end.
12 Programme your mind to be expansive and creative and eliminate the words 'I can't' from your vocabulary.
13 Learn to listen to others who have the benefit of experience and knowledge, and allow them to help you broaden your horizons.
14 Learn to accept that if you overindulge in your eating, this is, in itself, not a disaster. It just slows down your progress. If you continue with the diet plan, the indiscretion will work its way out over the next day or two.
15 For the first time, you actually feel in control of your eating and your body. It is a wonderful relief from previous feelings of guilt and restriction.
16 For the first time in your life you actually KNOW that you are a winner. You are not going to be a loser ever again.

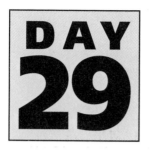

DAY 29
Continuing on the Programme

Congratulations! You've completed your 28-day plan and it's weighing and measuring time. Take a good look in the mirror. Look at your 'before' photograph. See the improvement.

If you still want to lose more weight and inches, you have the choice of either retracking your steps over the previous 28 days and following the menu plans that were designed for the first month, or you can make up your own menu plan from these same menus.

As before, always select one breakfast, lunch and dinner menu for each day, and remember your daily allowance of 150ml (¼ pint) unsweetened fruit juice, 450ml (¾ pint) skimmed or semi-skimmed milk, and that 1 measure of alcohol is permitted for women, 2 for men. On the first day of each new week that follows a full dieting week you are allowed an extra alcoholic drink to celebrate your achievement!

When selecting these menus, as a general rule please try to limit your intake of eggs to a maximum of 2 a week (vegetarians can have 3). Also remember that you can eat your main meal at lunchtime if you wish and have the snack meal in the evening. This is certainly recommended on the day prior to your weighing and measuring session. Try to eat a balanced diet that contains a good cross-section of nutrients.

It is important to eat two helpings of protein foods each day. You won't go short on vitamins and minerals because of the way the diet is designed, with plenty of fruit and vegetables and lots of carbohydrate recommended. Also, there is sufficient calcium to give you an adequate supply, and you will take in sufficient dietary fat from the foods that are included so there is no necessity to take it in additional forms. You should only take a dietary supplement if there is one particular group of foods that you are unable to eat for some reason. You can always consult your doctor or chemist for advice on this matter. I do, however, recommend that everyone takes a daily multi-vitamin tablet.

If you have yet to complete the programme of daily exercises, continue with the 28-day plan. Once you have mastered all of those you can simply continue to follow the exercises from Day 28 of the programme. Or you can follow the warm-up and aerobic sections from Day 28 and then choose your own toning exercises to focus on any particular areas of your body that you feel need further work.

When you have achieved the weight and inch loss you desire, please follow the Maintenance Eating Programme. Combine this with the exercises from Day 28 to see ongoing benefits to your shape and fitness.

Recipes

APPLE AND BLACKCURRANT WHIP

Serves 4

450g (1lb) cooking apples
50ml (2fl oz) water
saccharin or liquid artificial sweetener to taste
2 egg whites
2 tablespoons low-calorie blackcurrant jam or 115g
   (4oz) fresh or frozen blackcurrants

Peel, core and slice the apples and cook in the water until they become a thick pulp. Add saccharin or liquid artificial sweetener to taste. Set aside to cool.

Whisk the egg whites until stiff and gently fold into the cooked apple purée. Pile the mixture into individual sundae dishes or a medium-sized serving dish. Swirl the jam or blackcurrants on the top to give a ripple effect.

APRICOT PLUM SOFTIE

Serves 4

50g (2oz) fresh stoned dates
175g (6oz) fresh or 'no soak' apricots
275g (10oz) thick low-fat natural yogurt
2 egg whites
2 tablespoons Canderel
2 plums or apricots and a few sprigs of mint to
   decorate

Blend the dates and apricots with the yogurt in a food processor or liquidiser until smooth.

Whisk the egg whites until stiff and fold in the Canderel.

Carefully fold the date mixture into the egg white, and spoon into 4 serving dishes. Leave to set.

Just before serving, decorate with plum or apricot slices and mint.

AUTUMN PUDDING

Serves 6–8

7–9 thick slices white or brown bread
450–900g (1–2lb) mixed Autumn fruits (apples,
   pears, blackberries)
4 tablespoons water
5–6 tablespoons Canderel

Cut off the bread crusts and line the base and sides of a 1.2 litre (2 pint) pudding basin, reserving 2 slices for the top.

Prepare the fruit; peel, core and slice the apples and pears and hull the blackberries. Place the apple and pear slices in a saucepan. Add the water, cover with a tight-fitting lid and cook over a very gentle heat until just soft but not mushy. Remove from the heat and leave to cool.

Stir in the Canderel and the hulled blackberries. Using a slotted draining spoon, transfer the prepared fruit into the bread-lined basin. Add the remaining slices of bread. Cover with a piece of greaseproof paper, then place a saucer on top. Weight the saucer to encourage the juices from the fruit to soak into the bread. Refrigerate the pudding and remaining sauce overnight.

To serve, invert the basin on to a plate and pour the sauce over the pudding just before serving.

BAKED APPLES WITH APRICOTS

Serves 4

8–12 'no soak' apricots
2 tablespoons caster sugar, or artificial sweetener
   to taste
2 tablespoons rum
4 large dessert apples
1–2 tablespoons lemon juice
1 quantity of Apricot Sauce (see next recipe)

Wash the apricots and cut into small pieces. Place in a bowl with 1 teaspoon of sugar and the 2 table-spooons of rum. Leave to stand for 1 hour.

Peel the apples, leaving the stalks in place. Cut a slice (or lid) off the top of each apple and reserve. Using an apple corer or a small sharp knife, core the apples and place in an ovenproof dish.

Using a slotted spoon, lift the prepared apricots out of the rum and divide them between the 4 apples. Place the apricots in the centre of each apple and replace the lids. Brush with the lemon juice and pour the rum from the apricots over them. Sprinkle 1 teaspoon of sugar (if using) over the top of each apple. Pour 150ml (¼ pint) water into the dish.

Bake in a preheated oven at 200°C, 400°F, or Gas Mark 6 for 30–45 minutes. The apples must be cooked through but take care they don't fall apart. Halfway through the cooking time baste them with the juice and sprinkle a little more sugar or sweetener on each.

Meanwhile make the Apricot Sauce.

Heat the sauce, pour a little over each apple and serve the rest of the sauce separately.

APRICOT SAUCE

Serves 4–6

225g (8oz) 'no soak' apricots or 1 × 400g (14oz) tin
  apricots in natural juice
caster sugar or artificial sweetener to taste
2–3 tablespoons rum (optional)

Place the apricots in a pan with 175ml (6fl oz) of water. Cook over a gentle heat until tender (approx. 15–20 minutes).

Purée the stewed or tinned apricots with their juice in a food processor or liquidiser until smooth. Add the sugar or artificial sweetener to taste. Stir in the rum, if using.

Serve hot or cold.

BAKED STUFFED APPLE

Serves 1

25g (1oz) dried fruit
1 large apple, cored
1 teaspoon honey
2 tablespoons low-fat natural yogurt

Mix together the dried fruit and the honey. Pile into the centre of the apple. Bake in a moderate oven (200°C, 400°F, Gas Mark 6) for about half an hour.

Serve with the yogurt.

BARBECUED CHICKEN KEBABS

Serves 2

2 large boned chicken joints, preferably breasts, with
  all fat and skin removed
2 medium onions, peeled and quartered
1 green pepper, seeded and cut into bite-sized squares
1 red pepper, seeded and cut into bite-sized squares
175g (6oz) mushrooms, washed but left whole
8 bay leaves

for the barbecue sauce
2 tablespoons tomato ketchup
2 tablespoons brown sauce
2 tablespoons mushroom sauce (optional)
2 tablespoons wine vinegar

Cut the chicken into cubes. Thread the chicken cubes onto 2 small or 4 large skewers alternately with bite-sized pieces of onion, green and red peppers and mushrooms, placing a bay leaf on the skewers at intervals to add flavour.

Mix all the sauce ingredients together and brush onto the skewered chicken and vegetables. If possible, brush the sauce on a couple of hours before cooking as this will add to the flavour. Keep any remaining sauce for basting.

Place under the grill and cook under a moderate to high heat, basting frequently with the remaining sauce and turning regularly to avoid burning.

Serve on a bed of rice (use 150g/5oz cooked weight per person) and grilled fresh tomatoes.

BARBECUED VEGETABLE KEBABS

Serves 2

2 medium onions, peeled and quartered
1 green pepper, seeded and cut into bite-sized squares
1 red pepper, seeded and cut into bite-sized squares
175g (6oz) mushrooms, washed but left whole
4 medium firm tomatoes, halved crossways
8 bay leaves

for the barbecue sauce
2 tablespoons ketchup
2 tablespoons brown sauce
2 tablespoons mushroom sauce (optional)
2 tablespoons wine vinegar

Thread bite-sized pieces of onion, green and red peppers, mushrooms and tomatoes alternately onto 2 large or 4 small skewers, placing a bay leaf on the skewers at intervals to add flavour.

Mix all the sauce ingredients together and brush onto the skewered vegetables. If possible, brush the sauce on a couple of hours before cooking as this will add to the flavour. Keep any remaining sauce for basting.

Place the skewers under the grill and cook under a moderate heat, basting frequently with the remaining sauce and turning regularly to avoid burning.

Serve on a bed of rice (150g/5oz cooked weight per person), grilled fresh tomatoes and minted natural yogurt.

BLACKEYE BEAN CASSEROLE

Serves 2

50g (2oz) blackeye beans
50g (2oz) diced onions
175g (6oz) sliced mushrooms
115g (4oz) celery, cut into thin strips
75g (3oz) carrots, cut into thin strips
50g (2oz) water chestnuts, thinly sliced
1/2 teaspoon chilli
1/2 teaspoon grated fresh ginger or 1/2 teaspoon grated
  ginger
1 garlic clove, crushed
15g (1/2oz) cornflour
1 tablespoon soy sauce
150ml (1/4 pint) vegetable stock
freshly ground black pepper

Cook the blackeye beans in plenty of water for 30–35 minutes by bringing to the boil and then simmering in a covered pan. Drain.

Gently heat the vegetables, chilli, ginger and garlic in a little stock for 10 minutes. Mix the cornflour and soy sauce with a little stock and then stir in remainder of the stock. Add this mixture to the vegetables and then add the drained beans. Simmer for 8–10 minutes and season to taste.

Serve on a bed of boiled brown rice (150g/5oz cooked weight per person).

CARROT SALAD

Serves 1

2 large fresh carrots
25g (1oz) sultanas

Grate the carrots and mix with the sultanas. Serve with a salad or in a jacket potato.

CHEESE PEARS

Serves 1

1 ripe pear
lemon juice
50g (2oz) low-fat cottage cheese
1 teaspoon apricot jam or preserve

Peel and core the pear and cut in half lengthways. Brush with lemon juice to prevent discoloration.

Mix the cottage cheese with the jam or preserve and use to fill the cavities of the pear.

Serve chilled.

CHICKEN CHINESE-STYLE

Serves 4

4 chicken breasts, skinned
2 chicken stock cubes, mixed in 50ml (2fl oz) hot
  water
1 tablespoon soy sauce
1 onion, chopped
freshly ground black pepper
2 teaspoons cornflour mixed in 3 tablespoons water
500g (1¼lb) cooked weight boiled brown rice
  (prepared in advance)
1 × 400g (14oz) tin beansprouts, drained

Sauté the chicken breasts in a heavy-based non-stick frying pan until they change colour. Reduce the heat and add the water and stock cubes, soy sauce and chopped onion. Season well with plenty of freshly ground black pepper. Cover with a lid and simmer on a low heat for 15–20 minutes, stirring occasionally.

When the chicken is thoroughly cooked remove the breasts, place them on a preheated serving dish and keep warm.

Add the cornflour mixture into the frying pan and thicken to a creamy consistency. Take care to keep it on a low heat, as overheating at this stage may cause the sauce to go lumpy. If it thickens too quickly, remove from the heat immediately and stir vigorously. Add more water if necessary. When cooked, pour the sauce over the chicken breasts.

Mix the cooked rice and the beansprouts together in a large bowl. Heat the mixture thoroughly by placing it in a large colander and rinsing with plenty of boiling water. This method of reheating prevents overcooking.

Serve with additional soy sauce and unlimited vegetables of your choice.

CHICKEN CHOP SUEY

Serves 1

Vegetarians can follow this recipe and omit the chicken.

1 chicken joint, skinned and boned
1 tablespoon vegetable stock
1 large carrot, peeled and coarsely grated
1 large onion, finely sliced
2 celery sticks, finely chopped
1 green pepper, seeded and sliced
1 × 400g (14oz) tin beansprouts, drained
salt and pepper to taste
soy sauce

Coarsely slice the chicken, add to the vegetable stock and cook in a large non-stick frying pan or wok on a moderate heat until the chicken changes colour.

Add the grated carrot, sliced onion and chopped celery, and stir-fry.

Add the sliced green pepper and beansprouts and continue to cook until thoroughly hot. Season to taste. Serve on a bed of boiled brown rice (150g/5oz cooked weight per person) with soy sauce.

CHICKPEA AND FENNEL CASSEROLE

Serves 2

75g (3oz) cooked chickpeas
25g (1oz) bulgar wheat
175g (6oz) diced celery
2 teaspoons crushed fennel seeds
1 garlic clove, crushed
175g (6oz) whole green beans, chopped
300ml (½ pint) vegetable stock
2 tablespoons soy sauce
salt and freshly ground black pepper
2 tablespoons chopped fresh mint

Cook the chickpeas, bulgar wheat, celery, fennel and garlic gently in a little stock for about 5 minutes. Add the remaining ingredients excluding the mint.

Simmer for 20 minutes and serve with fresh mint and unlimited vegetables or boiled brown rice (150g/5oz cooked weight per person).

CHOCOLATE AND COFFEE ROULADE

Serves 6

2 eggs
2 tablespoons Canderel
40g (1½oz) plain flour
1 teaspoon cocoa powder
1 tablespoon coffee essence
1 tablespoon warm water

for the filling

150g (5oz) low-fat natural fromage frais mixed with 1 teaspoon Canderel

Line a small Swiss-roll tin (18 × 28cm/7 × 11in) with parchment paper. Whisk the eggs and Canderel together until very thick, fluffy and pale in colour. The mixture should leave a trail if the whisk is lifted out of the mixture for 4–5 seconds. Fold in the flour and cocoa powder along with the coffee and water. Bake at 200°C, 400°F, or Gas Mark 6 for about 10–12 minutes.

When cooked, turn out onto a clean piece of parchment paper. Trim about 5mm ($^1/_4$in) off each edge and quickly roll up the roll loosely with the parchment paper.

Mix all the filling ingredients together. When the 'cake' is cool, unroll it, remove the paper and spread the 'cake' with the filling, then re-roll it. Cut into slices and serve with fresh fruit if desired.

Note If you can't find parchment paper, use very lightly greased greaseproof paper.

COEURS A LA CREME

Serves 4

275g (10oz) low-fat natural fromage frais
1 tablespoon Canderel
115g (4oz) low-fat cottage cheese
4 whole raspberries and 4 sprigs of mint to decorate

for the sauce
275g (10oz) fresh or frozen raspberries
1–3 tablespoons Canderel or to taste

In a mixing bowl beat together the fromage frais, Canderel and cottage cheese until smooth.

Line 4 heart-shaped moulds or round biscuit-cutters (7.5cm/3in) with clean muslin. Spoon the cheese mixture into the moulds and smooth over the tops. Place the moulds onto a baking tray and leave to drain overnight in the refrigerator.

Invert onto 4 serving plates, then carefully remove the muslin and pour the raspberry sauce around each heart. Decorate with the raspberries and mint.

To make the sauce, rub the raspberries through a nylon sieve and mix in the Canderel.

COLESLAW

Serves 4

225g (8oz) white cabbage, trimmed
225g (8oz) carrots, peeled
$^1/_2$ Spanish onion
150g (5oz) reduced-oil salad dressing
salt and pepper

Grate the cabbage, carrots and onion, or chop in a food processor, and mix with the dressing. Season and keep chilled.

CURRIED CHICKEN AND YOGURT SALAD

Serves 1

1 × 150g (5oz) carton low-fat natural yogurt
1 teaspoon curry powder
50g (2oz) cooked chicken breast, cut into cubes
unlimited green salad and vegetables

Mix the yogurt and curry powder together and stir in cubes of cooked chicken.

Serve on a bed of fresh green salad vegetables.

DRY-ROAST POTATOES

Serves 3

450g (1lb) medium potatoes
salt

Peel the potatoes and cut into even-sized pieces if you wish. Place in a pan of cold water with a vegetable stock cube, bring to the boil and blanch for 5 minutes.

Drain thoroughly and place on a non-stick baking tray without any fat. Sprinkle lightly with salt and bake at the top in a preheated oven at 180°C, 350°F, or Gas Mark 4 for about 1 hour.

FISH CAKES

Serves 2

225g (8oz) cod, steamed
225g (8oz) potatoes, cooked
1 egg white
2 tablespoons finely chopped fresh parsley
1 teaspoon prepared mustard

Mash together the cod and potatoes. Add the egg white and stir well, then add the parsley and mustard. Wet your hands and form the mixture into fish cakes.

Dry-fry in a non-stick frying pan until golden brown on each side.

Serve with unlimited vegetables.

FISH CURRY

Serves 2

1 × 400g (14oz) tin tomatoes
1 bay leaf
1 eating apple, cored and chopped small
2 teaspoons Branston pickle
1 teaspoon of tomato purée
1 medium onion, finely chopped
1 tablespoon curry powder
2 pieces haddock or cod (approx. 450g/1lb total weight), cut into cubes

Place all the ingredients except the fish in a saucepan, and bring to the boil. Put a lid on the saucepan and cook slowly for about 1 hour, stirring occasionally.

Approximately 20 minutes before the end of cooking time, add the fish to the saucepan. If the mixture is too thin, remove the lid and cook on a slightly higher heat until the sauce reduces and thickens towards the end of the cooking time.

Serve on a bed of boiled brown rice (150g/5oz cooked weight per person).

FISH KEBABS

Serves 2

350g (12oz) white fish (thick flesh), cut into bite-
    sized pieces
1 green pepper, seeded and chopped into 2cm (¾in)
    squares
1 red pepper, seeded and chopped into 2cm (¾in)
    squares
1 large Spanish onion, peeled and cut into large
    pieces, or 175g (6oz) small button onions, peeled
225g (8oz) button mushrooms, washed
450g (1lb) medium tomatoes, sliced across sideways
1 teaspoon mixed herbs
1 tablespoon wine vinegar
freshly ground black pepper
115g (4oz) cooked sweetcorn
115g (4oz) cooked brown rice

Preheat the oven to 180°C, 350°F, or Gas Mark 4.
Thread the fish cubes and vegetable pieces alternately
onto 4 skewers to make 4 kebabs.

Cover a baking tray with foil and place the kebabs
on the foil. Sprinkle each kebab with the herbs, wine
vinegar and pepper. Wrap the foil around the kebabs
to make a parcel and cook for 30 minutes.

Remove from oven. Place on a bed of hot
sweetcorn and rice.

Replace in the oven for 1 minute.

FISH PIE

Serves 4

675g (1½lb) cod
675g (1½lb) potatoes
salt and pepper
50g (2oz) grated low-fat Cheddar cheese (optional,
    for maintenance dieters only)

Bake, steam or microwave the fish but do not
overcook. Season well.

Boil the potatoes until well done and mash with
a little water and milk to make a soft consistency.
Season well.

Place the fish in an ovenproof dish, flake the
flesh, remove the skin, and distribute the fish evenly
across the base of the dish.

Cover the fish completely with the mashed potatoes and smooth over with a fork. Sprinkle the cheese
on the top (if using).

If the ingredients are still hot, just place under a
hot grill for a few minutes to brown the top.
Alternatively you can make the pie well in advance
and then warm it through in a preheated moderate
oven (180°C, 350°F, Gas Mark 4) for 20 minutes.

FISH RISOTTO

Serves 4

For special occasions you could add prawns and
green peppers to this dish.

3 frozen haddock fillets
4 tablespoons brown rice
1 medium onion, chopped
50g (2oz) mushrooms, sliced
1 × 200g (7oz) tin chopped tomatoes
1 teaspoon oregano
salt and black pepper
1 glass of white wine
50g (2oz) frozen peas
25g (1oz) grated low-fat Cheddar cheese (optional,
    for maintenance dieters only)

Poach the fish in the water until it is cooked. Remove
the skin and break the flesh into chunks.

Meanwhile, cook the rice in salted water. As soon
as the rice is simmering, add the chopped onion.
When the rice is half-cooked, add the mushrooms,
tomatoes, oregano and pepper. Next add the wine
and the frozen peas.

When almost all the liquid has evaporated, add

the fish. Just before serving, sprinkle with the cheese
(if using).

FRUITY APPLE TERRINE

Serves 6–8

450ml (¾ pint) unsweetened apple or orange juice
1 packet powdered gelatine dissolved in 3
    tablespoons water
3 tablespoons Canderel
assortment of seasonal fruits, e.g. oranges, bananas,
    apples, peaches, strawberries, seedless grapes

Rinse a 675g (1½lb) non-stick loaf tin with cold
water. Mix the apple juice with the dissolved gelatine
and Canderel. Pour a thin layer into the tin and leave
to set in the refrigerator.

Prepare the fruit: peel and slice the oranges and
bananas; peel and core the apples and cut into slices;
peel the peaches and cut into slices; hull the
raspberries.

Make a pretty pattern, using the grapes and the
banana slices. Carefully pour a little apple jelly over
them and leave to set.

Continue arranging different layers of fruit and
setting each layer with the apple jelly before adding
another. Make sure that the last layer of fruit is completely covered with apple jelly. Leave to set overnight
in the refrigerator.

To serve, dip the loaf tin quickly into hot water
and invert onto a serving plate. Cut into slices and
serve each slice with 1 tablespoon of low-fat fromage
frais or diet yogurt.

GARLIC MUSHROOMS

Serves 4

450g (1lb) button mushrooms
300ml (½ pint) chicken stock
3 garlic cloves, crushed
salt and pepper

Wash the mushrooms and drain.

Place the chicken stock and garlic in a saucepan. Boil for 5 minutes on a gentle heat. Add the mushrooms, place a lid on the pan, and simmer for a further 7 minutes.

Serve in soup dishes.

HOME-MADE MUESLI

Serves 1

15g ($^1/_2$oz) oats
15g ($^1/_2$oz) sultanas or $^1/_2$ banana
2 teaspoons bran
1 eating apple, grated or chopped
milk from allowance mixed with 75g (3oz) low-fat
    natural yogurt
honey to taste (optional)

Mix all the ingredients together and add honey to taste if desired.

Alternatively mix all the dry ingredients (except the banana) the night before and leave to soak in skimmed milk.

HOT CHERRIES

Serves 2

small tin black cherries
50ml (2fl oz) cherry brandy (optional)
1 teaspoon slaked arrowroot
50g (2oz) Wall's 'Too Good To Be True' frozen dessert

Strain the cherries, reserving the juice. Heat the juice in a pan, add the cherry brandy, if using, and thicken with sufficient slaked arrowroot (approx. 1 teaspoon of arrowroot mixed with water) to make a syrup.

Pour the syrup over the frozen dessert and serve immediately with the cherries.

INCH LOSS SALAD

Serves 1

unlimited amounts of shredded lettuce, chopped
    cucumber and any other green salad
1 apple
1 kiwi fruit
1 orange
1 pear
50g (2oz) chicken or prawns
75g (3oz) low-fat natural yogurt
1 tablespoon wine vinegar
1 garlic clove, crushed
salt and freshly ground black pepper

Place the lettuce and green salad on a large dinner plate. Lay slices of the various fruits around the dish and place the chopped chicken or prawns in the centre.

Make up a dressing with the yogurt, wine vinegar and garlic and season to taste. Serve with the salad.

KIM'S CAKE

1 serving = 1cm/$^1/_2$in slice

For a special occasion you could add some cherries in addition to the dried fruit.

450g (1lb) mixed dried fruit
1 mug soft brown sugar
2 mugs self-raising flour
1 beaten egg

Soak the dried fruit overnight in a mug of hot black tea. Mix all ingredients together and place in a loaf tin or round cake tin. Bake for 2 hours at 160°C, 325°F, or Gas Mark 3.

LENTIL ROAST

Serves 3–4

350g (12oz) orange lentils
1 bay leaf
2–3 parsley stalks
1 sprig fresh thyme
2 large onions
1–2 garlic cloves
2–3 celery sticks
$^1/_2$ green pepper
$^1/_2$ red pepper
1 dessert apple
75g (3oz) plain low-fat quark or fromage frais or
    yogurt
salt and freshly ground black pepper

Wash the lentils well, drain and place in a large pan. Cover with water. (Do not add salt at this stage.) Tie the bay leaf, parsley stalks and thyme together with string and add to the pan. Bring to the boil.

Peel the onions and garlic. Chop the onion and crush the garlic. Wash, trim and slice the celery. Add the onions, garlic and celery to the lentils and simmer until the lentils and vegetables are tender and the liquid has almost evaporated.

Remove the pith and seeds from the peppers. Peel the apple, cut into quarters and remove the core. Cut both the peppers and the apple into small dice.

When the lentils are tender, remove the bunch of herbs and continue cooking, stirring all the time until the mixture is quite dry. Stir in the peppers and apples and add the quark. Mix well and season to taste with salt and freshly ground black pepper.

Pile the mixture into an ovenproof dish or loaf tin and bake in a preheated oven at 180°C, 350°F, or Gas Mark 4 for about 1 hour until the top is springy like a sponge.

Serve with a selection of seasonal vegetables.

MELON SURPRISE

Serves 1

225g (8oz) melon flesh
1 × 150g (5oz) diet yogurt, any flavour

Finely chop the melon flesh and mix with the diet yogurt. Serve chilled.

OATY YOGURT DESSERT

Serves 4

2 dessert apples
50g (2oz) seedless raisins
275g (10oz) low-fat natural yogurt
4 tablespoons porridge oats
2 tablespoons golden syrup or honey
4 glacé cherries
small piece of angelica

Peel, core and finely chop the apples. Coarsely chop the raisins.

Place the yogurt in a bowl and add the chopped apples, raisins, porridge oats and golden syrup or honey. Mix thoroughly.

Spoon the mixture into individual glasses, cover with clingfilm and refrigerate for 3–4 hours.

Decorate each glass with a glacé cherry and leaves cut from the angelica. Serve chilled.

OIL-FREE ORANGE AND LEMON VINAIGRETTE DRESSING

120ml (4fl oz) wine vinegar
4 tablespoons lemon juice
4 tablespoons orange juice
grated rind of 1 lemon
$1/2$ teaspoon French mustard
pinch of garlic salt
freshly ground black pepper

Place all the ingredients in a bowl and mix thoroughly. Keep in the refrigerator and use within 2 days.

ORANGE AND CARROT SALAD

Serves 1

1 large orange
green salad vegetables (e.g. cucumber, onion, cabbage, chicory, endives)
115g (4oz) low-fat cottage cheese
115g (4oz) grated carrot

Remove the peel and pith from the orange and slice the flesh into rounds.

Arrange the orange flesh on a bed of chopped green salad vegetables. Place the cottage cheese in the centre and pile the grated carrot on top.

Dress with OIL-FREE ORANGE AND LEMON VINAIGRETTE DRESSING (see previous recipe).

ORANGES IN COINTREAU

Serves 4

1 wine glass of medium to sweet white wine or fresh orange juice
1 sherry glass of Cointreau or Grand Marnier liqueur
artificial sweetener to taste (optional)
6 medium oranges

Heat the white wine or orange juice and the liqueur in a saucepan and add sweetener to taste. Allow to cool.

Carefully peel the oranges with a sharp knife to remove all pith. This can be done by slicing the peel across the top of the orange and then using the flat end of the orange as a base. Cut strips of peel away from the top downwards with a very sharp knife so that the orange is completely free from the white membranes of the peel. Squeeze the peel to extract any juice and pour this into the wine mixture.

Slice the oranges across to form round slices of equal size. When the liquid is cool add to the oranges.

Allow to stand in a refrigerator for at least 12 hours. Serve in glass dishes with fromage frais.

OVEN CHIPS

Serves 4

2–3 large potatoes
1 teaspoon oil

Peel the potatoes and cut into chips. Blanch in boiling water with a vegetable stock cube for 5 minutes, then drain well.

Meanwhile, brush the oil onto a baking sheet and place in a preheated oven at 220°C, 425°F, or Gas Mark 7 for 7–10 minutes until the oil is very hot.

Spread the chips over the baking tray and turn them gently so that they are lightly coated with oil. Bake for 35–40 minutes (depending on the size of the chips) until they are soft in the middle and crisp on the outside. Turn them once or twice during the cooking time.

PARSLEY SAUCE

Serves 4

300ml ($1/2$ pint) skimmed milk
2 teaspoons cornflour
1 onion, peeled and sliced
6 peppercorns
1 bay leaf
chopped fresh parsley
salt and freshly ground black pepper

Place all but 50ml (2fl oz) of the milk in a non-stick saucepan. Add the onion, peppercorns, bay leaf and seasoning. Cover the pan and heat gently. Simmer for 5 minutes. Turn off the heat and leave the milk mixture to stand, with the lid on, for a further 30 minutes or until you are ready to thicken and serve the sauce.

Mix the remaining milk with cornflour and, when almost ready to serve, strain the seasoned milk, add the cornflour mixture and reheat slowly, stirring continuously, until it comes to the boil. Add the freshly chopped parsley. If the sauce begins to thicken too quickly, remove from the heat and stir very fast to mix well. Cook for 3–4 minutes and serve immediately.

PEARS IN MERINGUE

Serves 6

6 ripe dessert pears, peeled but left whole
300ml (1/2 pint) apple juice
3 egg whites
175g (6oz) caster sugar

Cook the pears in the apple juice until just tender.

Cut a slice off the bottom of each pear to enable them to sit in a dish without falling over. Place them, well spaced out, in an ovenproof dish.

Whisk the egg whites in a large and completely grease-free bowl, preferably with a balloon whisk or rotary beater, as these make more volume than an electric whisk.

When the egg whites are firm and stand in peaks, whisk in 1 tablespoon of caster sugar for 1 minute. Fold in the remainder of the sugar with a metal spoon, cutting the egg whites rather than mixing them.

Place the egg white and sugar mixture into a large piping bag with a metal nozzle (any pattern) and pipe a pyramid around each pear, starting from the base and working upwards. Place in a moderate oven at 160°C, 325°F, or Gas Mark 3 and cook until firm and golden.

Serve hot or cold.

PEARS IN RED WINE

Serves 4

6 ripe pears, peeled but left whole
50g (2oz) brown sugar
2 wine glasses of red wine
50ml (2fl oz) water
1/2 level teaspoon cinnamon or ground ginger

To microwave
Combine the wine, water, sugar and spice in a glass jug and microwave on High for approximately 4 minutes or until boiling.

Place the pears in a deep soufflé dish, pour the wine sauce over and cover with clingfilm. Microwave on High for approximately 5 minutes or until they are just tender but retain their shape.

To cook on the stove
Combine the wine, water, sugar and spice in a large saucepan and bring to the boil. Add the pears to the pan and simmer for 10–15 minutes, turning the pears carefully from time to time to ensure even colouring.

Serve hot or cold with fromage frais.

PINEAPPLE AND ORANGE SORBET

Serves 6

1 small tin crushed pineapple in natural juice
1 orange, peeled and chopped
250ml (8fl oz) fresh orange juice
Canderel to taste
2 egg whites

Crush the pineapple well and mix with the chopped orange and the orange juice. Sweeten to taste. Place in a plastic container in the freezer or in the freezer compartment of the refrigerator. Freeze until half-frozen, then remove from the freezer and work a fork through the mixture to make it softer.

Whisk the egg whites until stiff. Turn out the half-frozen mixture into a bowl and fold in the whisked egg whites. Return mixture to the freezer until firm.

PINEAPPLE BOAT

Serves 2

1 medium fresh pineapple
225g (8oz) seasonal fruit of your choice
150g (5oz) diet yogurt, any flavour
2 cherries or strawberries to decorate

Divide the pineapple into 2 halves from top to bottom. Do not cut away the leaves, as they add to the decorative look. Cut away the flesh with a grapefruit knife and cut this flesh into cubes, removing the hard core.

Prepare the remaining fruit: wash and cut it into bite-sized pieces and mix with the pineapple flesh. Pile into the hollowed-out pineapple halves and dress with the yogurt.

Serve chilled and decorate each half with either a cherry or strawberry.

PINEAPPLE IN KIRSCH

Serves 4

1 fresh pineapple
1 liqueur or sherry glass of Kirsch

Remove the skin and core from the pineapple and slice into rings. Sprinkle the Kirsch over the fruit and place in a refrigerator for at least 12 hours to marinate. Keep turning the fruit to ensure even flavouring.

PINEAPPLE SAUCE

Serves 2

1 large cooking apple, cooked to a pulp
250ml (8fl oz) natural pineapple juice
Canderel to taste

Mix the apple purée and pineapple juice together and sweeten to taste. Heat gently in a saucepan. When hot, serve in a sauce boat. If the sauce is too thick, you can add more juice.

PORRIDGE

Serves 1

25g (1oz) porridge oats
300ml (1/2 pint) water
2 teaspoons liquid honey

Place the porridge oats and the cold water in a small milk saucepan and heat gently until boiling. Leave covered overnight.

Stir well and reheat until thoroughly hot. To serve, pour milk from your allowance into a cereal dish, tip the porridge into this and it will float. Now pour the 2 teaspoons of liquid honey onto the porridge.

PRAWN CURRY

Serves 2

225g (8oz) fresh or frozen prawns
1 × 400g (14oz) tin tomatoes
bay leaf
1 eating apple cored and chopped small
2 teaspoons Branston pickle
1 teaspoon tomato purée
1 medium onion, finely chopped
50g (2oz) frozen peas
1 tablespoon curry powder

If using frozen prawns, allow them to thaw completely.

Place all the ingredients except the prawns in a saucepan and bring to the boil. Put a lid on the saucepan and cook slowly for about 1 hour, stirring occasionally.

Approximately 10 minutes before the end of cooking time, add the prawns to the saucepan. If the mixture is too thin, remove the lid and cook on a slightly higher heat until the sauce reduces and thickens.

Serve on a bed of boiled brown rice (150g/5oz cooked weight per person).

RASPBERRY & STRAWBERRY BAVAROIS

Serves 4

2 egg yolks
175ml (6fl oz) skimmed milk
3 tablespoons Canderel

15g (1/2oz) powdered gelatine dissolved in 4 tablespoons hot water
2 tablespoons thick low-fat natural yogurt
few drops of vanilla essence
225g (8oz) fresh or frozen raspberries and/or strawberries, lightly crushed
a few fresh raspberry or mint leaves to decorate

for the sauce

225g (8oz) fresh or frozen raspberries and/or strawberries, roughly chopped
1–2 tablespoons Canderel

Mix the egg yolks with the milk. Cook over a gentle heat until the mixture just coats the back of a wooden spoon. Take off the heat and allow to cool. When cold, add the Canderel, gelatine, yogurt and vanilla essence. Just before setting, fold in the fruit and pour into a ring mould. Leave to chill in the refrigerator.

Make the sauce by pushing half the sauce fruit through a nylon sieve and sweeten to taste with the Canderel.

Invert the bavarois onto a serving plate, pour the sauce around the base of the plate and fill the middle with the remaining fruit. Decorate with raspberry or mint leaves and a sprinkling of Canderel.

RASPBERRY FLUFF

Serves 4

225g (8oz) fresh raspberries
1 egg white (optional) see note
50g (2oz) caster sugar
450g (1lb) low-fat fromage frais or low-fat yogurt

Wash the raspberries and drain well. Reserve a few for decoration and mash the rest slightly with a fork.

Whisk the egg white in a clean dry bowl until it stands in stiff peaks. Using a metal spoon or spatula, carefully fold in the sugar and then the fromage frais.

Layer the fromage frais and raspberries into 4 tall glasses, ending with a layer of fromage frais.

Decorate the top with a few whole raspberries. Refrigerate until required.

Note If you prefer to avoid the use of uncooked egg white, omit it and just layer the fromage frais and raspberries.

RASPBERRY MOUSSE

Serves 4

225g (8oz) fresh raspberries or 200g (7oz) tinned raspberries in natural juice
120ml (4fl oz) natural apple juice
2 tablespoons caster sugar
1 teaspoon gelatine
2 egg whites
1 teaspoon low-fat natural yogurt or fromage frais
12 fresh raspberries to decorate

Place the raspberries and apple juice in a liquidiser and blend until smooth. Strain through a sieve into a basin and add the sugar.

Dissolve the gelatine in 3 teaspoons of water in a cup over very hot water. Stir into the raspberry purée.

Whisk the egg whites until they form peaks. Fold into the purée. Pour the mixture into tall sundae glasses or a serving dish, and chill.

Just before serving, decorate each glass with fresh raspberries and 1 teaspoon of yogurt or fromage frais.

RATATOUILLE

Serves 2

225g (8oz) courgettes
2 aubergines
1 large green pepper
2 small onions, finely sliced into rings
1 × 400g (14oz) tin tomatoes
2 garlic cloves, chopped (optional)
2 bay leaves
salt and freshly ground black pepper

Slice the courgettes and aubergines. Halve the pepper, remove the core and seeds, and cut the flesh into fine strips.

Place the vegetables and the tinned tomatoes in a large saucepan, and add the remaining ingredients. Bring to the boil and skim off any sediment if necessary. Cover and simmer for about 20 minutes or until all vegetables are tender. If there is too much liquid remaining, reduce this by boiling it briskly for a few minutes with the lid removed.

Note Ratatouille can also be used as a main course if accompanied by 175g (6oz) chicken or 225g (8oz) white fish (cooked weights).

RICE SALAD

Serves 1

1 green pepper, seeded and cored
1 tomato
5cm (2in) piece of cucumber
50g (2oz) boiled brown rice, rinsed and drained
25g (1oz) cooked peas
25g (1oz) cooked sweetcorn
soy sauce
black pepper and pinch of salt

Chop the pepper, cucumber and tomato very finely and mix in with the rice, peas and sweetcorn. Add the soy sauce, and season to taste.

SALAD SURPRISE

Serves 1

115g (4oz) low-fat cottage cheese
1 tablespoon reduced-oil salad dressing
25g (1oz) cooked sweetcorn
unlimited chopped tomato, cucumber, spring onions, peppers
salt and black pepper

Mix all the ingredients together and season to taste.

SEAFOOD DRESSING

Serves 2

2 tablespoons tomato ketchup
1 tablespoon reduced-oil salad dressing
squeeze of lemon juice

Mix all the ingredients together and keep in the refrigerator for up to 2 days.

SHEPHERD'S PIE

Serves 4

450g (1lb) minced beef
300ml (½ pint) water
1 large onion, finely chopped
1 teaspoon mixed herbs
salt and freshly ground black pepper
1 teaspoon yeast or beef or vegetable extract (e.g. Marmite, Bovril)
3–4 teaspoons gravy powder
675g (1½lb) potatoes, peeled

Boil the mince and water in a saucepan for 5 minutes. Drain the mince and place in a covered container until required. Meanwhile, place the drained liquid in the refrigerator. This will cause any fat to rise to the top and set hard so that it can be removed and discarded.

Return the skimmed liquid to the saucepan. Add the mince, chopped onion, herbs, salt and pepper and yeast or beef extract. Mix the gravy powder with a little water and add to the meat mixture. Bring to the boil, stirring continuously and leave to simmer for a further 10 minutes.

Boil the potatoes until soft, then remove most but not all of the water, as the potatoes need to be quite wet for mashing. Mash the potatoes and season well, adding a little skimmed milk if necessary to make a soft consistency.

Place the mince in an oval ovenproof dish and cover with the mashed potatoes. Place under a hot grill to brown the top or in a preheated oven at 160°C, 325°F, or Gas Mark 3 for 10 minutes.

Serve with unlimited carrots and/or green vegetables.

SPAGHETTI BOLOGNESE

Serves 4

450g (1lb) lean mince
freshly ground black pepper
1 large onion, peeled and finely chopped
400g (14oz) tinned chopped tomatoes
75g (3oz) tomato purée
½ teaspoon oregano
2 garlic cloves, peeled and crushed
1 beef stock cube
200g (7oz) spaghetti

Heat a non-stick pan and, as you do so, sprinkle liberally with black pepper. Dry-fry the mince in the pan until the meat has changed colour and all the fat has liquified. Drain the mince through a sieve or colander and discard the fat.

Wipe out the pan with a paper towel, then return it to the heat. Add the onion and cook slowly until soft and slightly brown. Add the drained mince, chopped tomatoes, tomato purée, oregano and garlic and mix carefully. Cook on a medium heat for 15 minutes or until the meat is thoroughly cooked and the flavours absorbed.

Meanwhile, dissolve the stock cube in a pan of boiling water. Add the spaghetti and cook until just soft. Drain the spaghetti through a colander. Arrange the spaghetti on individual plates and pour the sauce on top.

SPICED BEAN CASSEROLE

Serves 2

50g (2oz) chopped onion
1 × 200g (7oz) tin tomatoes
³/₄ teaspoon mild chilli powder
¹/₂ teaspoon tomato purée
150ml (¹/₄ pint) vegetable stock
1 garlic clove, crushed
115g (4oz) sliced courgettes
175g (6oz) sliced red and green peppers
1 × 200g (7oz) tin red kidney beans, washed and
   drained
1 × 200g (7oz) tin haricot beans
115g (4oz) sweetcorn
25g (1oz) cornflour

Dry-fry the onion in a non-stick frying pan until soft. Add the tinned tomatoes, mild chilli powder, tomato purée and mix well.

Add all the remaining ingredients except the cornflour and bring to the boil.

Mix the cornflour with a little cold water and add to the mixture a little at a time until it is thickened slightly. Cover and simmer for 10–12 minutes or until the vegetables are tender.

Serve with mashed potatoes.

STIR-FRIED CHICKEN AND VEGETABLES

Serves 1

115g (4oz) chicken (no skin), coarsely sliced
1 × 400g (14oz) tin beansprouts, drained
3 celery sticks, washed and finely sliced
1 Spanish onion, peeled and finely sliced
75g (3oz) mushrooms, washed and sliced
75g (3oz) boiled brown rice

Partly cook the chicken in a non-stick frying pan or wok until it changes colour. Add the prepared vegetables a little at a time until all the ingredients are lightly cooked.

Serve with the rice.

STRAWBERRY WINE JELLY

Serves 4

225g (8oz) fresh strawberries
2 tablespoons brandy
475ml (16fl oz) rosé wine
1 tablespoon powdered gelatine dissolved in 3
   tablespoons hot water
2 tablespoons Canderel
4 whole strawberries and a few fresh strawberry leaves
   to decorate

Hull the strawberries and place in a bowl. Sprinkle the brandy over the top and leave for 30 minutes.

Pour the wine over the strawberries. Stir in the dissolved gelatine and the Canderel. Pour a little of the wine and fruit into 4 serving glasses and leave to set in the refrigerator.

Continue to add a little, each time leaving it to set, until it is all used up. This way, the fruit is suspended throughout the glass. Chill until set.

Decorate with the strawberries and strawberry leaves.

STUFFED MARROW

Serves 4

225g (8oz) assorted chopped vegetables
25g (1oz) chopped onion
2 garlic cloves, peeled and crushed
2 tablespoons tomato purée
2 teaspoons chopped fresh rosemary or 1 teaspoon
dried rosemary
salt and freshly ground black pepper
115g (4oz) uncooked weight long-grain brown rice
1 vegetable stock cube
1 medium marrow

Cook the vegetables, onion, garlic, tomato purée and rosemary in a little water seasoned with salt and pepper. Simmer until tender. Leave the mixture for the flavour to develop overnight.

Cook the rice in a saucepan of boiling water with a vegetable stock cube until tender.

Meanwhile, skin the marrow, cut it in half lengthways and remove the seeds.

When the rice is cooked, drain it, then mix it with the vegetable mixture. Spoon the mixture into the marrow halves. Wrap the stuffed marrow in foil and bake in a preheated oven at 200°C, 400°F, or Gas Mark 6 for 1 hour.

Serve with additional vegetables if desired.

STUFFED PEPPERS

Serves 1

2 red or green peppers
25g (1oz) uncooked weight brown rice
1 teaspoon mixed herbs
1 teaspoon sweetcorn
1 teaspoon peas
1 teaspoon chopped mushrooms
¹/₂ medium onion, chopped
salt and freshly ground black pepper

Wash the peppers, remove the tops, scoop out the core and seeds.

Boil the rice with the herbs until the rice is tender. Drain. Mix the rice and the remaining vegetables together. Add the seasoning and pile the mixture into the peppers. Place on a baking tray, and bake in a moderate oven (160°C, 325°F, Gas Mark 3) for 20 minutes.

Serve with additional unlimited vegetables and potatoes if desired.

SWEETCORN AND POTATO FRITTERS

Serves 2

225g (8oz) cooked potatoes
225g (8oz) cooked sweetcorn
1 egg white
2 tablespoons finely chopped fresh parsley
1 teaspoon prepared mustard

Mash the potatoes and mix with the cooked sweet-corn. Whisk the egg white and stir into the mixture. Add the parsley and the mustard.

Wet your hands and form the mixture into little cakes (approx. 6cm/2½in in diameter).

Dry-fry the cakes in a non-stick frying pan until golden brown on each side.

TRIPLE DECKER SANDWICH

Serves 1

3 slices bread
oil-free sweet pickle (e.g. Branston) or mustard
tomato ketchup
25g (1oz) wafer thin chicken or turkey
assorted salad ingredients (e.g. shredded lettuce,
   sliced tomato, cucumber and Spanish onion)
reduced-oil salad dressing
50g (2oz) low-fat cottage cheese

Spread 1 slice of bread with oil-free sweet pickle or mustard and another with ketchup. Place the chicken or turkey and some salad on the first slice and place the second slice on top to make a sandwich.

Spread the top side of the sandwich with reduced-oil salad dressing, top with the cottage cheese and remaining salad.

Spread the third slice of bread with reduced-oil salad dressing and place on top of the cottage cheese and salad.

VEGETABLE BAKE

Serves 1

selection of vegetables, e.g. carrots, parsnips, peas,
   cabbage, leeks, onions
1 teaspoon mixed herbs
3 tablespoons packet stuffing mix
115g (4oz) mushrooms
175g (6oz) cooked potatoes
1 cup breadcrumbs (preferably wholemeal)
300ml (½ pint) vegetable stock

Chop the assorted vegetables and cook until tender. Place the cooked vegetables in layers in a small ovenproof or microwave dish, sprinkling some mixed herbs and stuffing mix between each layer.

Slice the mushrooms and place on top of the vegetables in the dish. Slice the cooked potatoes and carefully lay them across the top of the dish, then sprinkle the breadcrumbs on top. Carefully pour the vegetable stock over to moisten the contents of the dish.

Bake in a moderate oven (180°C, 350°F, Gas Mark 4) for 20 minutes until piping hot. Alternatively, place in a microwave on High for 7 minutes, then place under a hot grill for 5 minutes to crisp the top.

VEGETABLE CURRY

Serves 4

75g (3oz) dry weight soya chunks
1 × 400g (14oz) tin tomatoes
1 bay leaf
1 eating apple, chopped
2 teaspoons Branston pickle
1 teaspoon tomato purée
1 medium onion, chopped
1 tablespoon curry powder

Soak the soya chunks in 2 cups of boiling water for 10 minutes. Drain.

Place the soya chunks and all the remaining ingredients in a saucepan and bring to the boil. Cover the saucepan and simmer for about 1 hour, stirring occasionally. If the mixture is too thin, remove the lid and cook on a slightly higher heat until the sauce reduces and thickens.

Serve on a bed of boiled brown rice (150g/5oz cooked weight per person).

VEGETABLE KEBABS

Serves 2

1 green and 1 red pepper, seeded and chopped into
   2cm (¾in) squares
1 large Spanish onion, cut into large pieces, or 175g
   (6oz) small button onions
225g (8oz) button mushrooms
4 courgettes, coarsely sliced
450g (1lb) medium tomatoes, cut in half
1 teaspoon thyme
275g (10oz) boiled brown rice (cooked weight)
cayenne pepper to taste

Thread the vegetable pieces alternately onto 4 skewers to make 4 kebabs.

Cover a baking sheet with foil and place the kebabs on the foil. Sprinkle each kebab with thyme. Wrap the foil around the kebabs to make a parcel and cook in a preheated oven at 180°C, 350°F, or Gas Mark 4 for 30 minutes.

Remove the kebabs from the oven. Place on a bed of rice, sprinkle with cayenne pepper then return to the oven for 1 minute.

VEGETABLE RISOTTO

Serves 2

4 tablespoons uncooked brown rice
1 medium onion, chopped
1 teaspoon oregano
1 green and 1 red pepper, seeded and finely chopped

50g (2oz) mushrooms, sliced
1 × 200g (7oz) tin chopped tomatoes
1 glass of white wine
50g (2oz) frozen peas
salt and black pepper
25g (1oz) grated half-fat Cheddar (optional, maintenance dieters only)

Place the rice in a saucepan of salted water and bring to the boil. As soon as the rice is simmering, add the chopped onion. When the rice is half-cooked, add the oregano, peppers, mushrooms and tomatoes. Next, add the wine and the frozen peas, and season to taste with salt and black pepper.

When cooked, sprinkle the cheese over the risotto and serve immediately.

VEGETARIAN CHILLI CON CARNE

Serves 4

75g (3oz) dry weight soya savoury mince
1 × 400g (14oz) tin chopped tomatoes
2 bay leaves
1 large onion, chopped
1 teaspoon yeast extract
1 × 400g (14oz) tin red kidney beans
1 teaspoon chilli powder or to taste
1 garlic clove, crushed (optional)

Pour 2 cups of boiling water on the soya mince and leave to stand for 10 minutes. Drain.

Place the soya and all the remaining ingredients in a saucepan, cover and cook for about 30 minutes. Towards the end of the cooking time, remove the lid and continue cooking until the mixture reaches a fairly thick consistency.

Serve with boiled brown rice (150g/5oz cooked weight per person).

VEGETARIAN GOULASH

Serves 2

75g (3oz) soya chunks
1 large onion, chopped
75g (3oz) carrots, sliced
75g (3oz) potato, cut into small chunks
1 × 400g (14oz) tin tomatoes
300ml (½ pint) vegetable stock
1 red pepper, seeded and chopped
2 bay leaves
2 teaspoons paprika
3 tablespoons low-fat natural yogurt
salt and pepper to taste

Pour 2 cups of boiling water on the soya chunks and leave to stand for 10 minutes. Drain.

Place the soya and all the remaining ingredients except the yogurt in a saucepan. Bring to the boil, cover and simmer for about 1 hour. Stir in the yogurt and season to taste.

Serve with boiled potatoes.

VEGETARIAN SHEPHERD'S PIE

Serves 4

75g (3oz) dry weight soya savoury mince
1 large onion, finely sliced
1 × 400g (14oz) tin chopped tomatoes
1 teaspoon mixed herbs
1 teaspoon yeast extract
120ml (4fl oz) vegetable stock
salt and freshly ground black pepper
1 tablespoon gravy powder mixed with a little water
675g (1½lb) potatoes, cooked and mashed (with water)

Pour 2 cups of boiling water over the soya and leave to stand for 10 minutes. Drain.

Place the soya mince, onion, tomatoes, herbs, yeast extract, vegetable stock and seasoning in a saucepan. Bring to the boil and simmer for 20 minutes. Add the gravy powder mixed with water and stir until the mixture thickens. Simmer uncovered for a further 5 minutes.

Place the mince mixture in an oval ovenproof dish and cover with the mashed potatoes. Place under a preheated grill to brown the top or in a preheated oven at 160°C, 325°F, or Gas Mark 3 for 10 minutes.

Serve with unlimited vegetables.

VEGETARIAN SPAGHETTI BOLOGNESE

Serves 4

75g (3oz) dry weight soya mince
75g (3oz) mushrooms
1 × 400g (14oz) tin chopped tomatoes
½ green pepper, seeded and finely chopped
1 teaspoon yeast extract
1 teaspoon oregano
2 garlic cloves, chopped
1 tablespoon gravy powder
275g (10oz) dry weight spaghetti

Pour 2 cups of boiling water on the soya and leave to stand for 10 minutes. Drain.

Place the soya mince, mushrooms, tomatoes, pepper, yeast extract, oregano and garlic in a saucepan. Cover and simmer for 20 minutes. Mix the gravy powder with a little cold water and stir into the sauce mixture.

Boil the spaghetti for 10–15 minutes until tender. Drain and place in a serving dish. Pour the sauce on top.

The Maintenance Programme

For most slimmers, actually losing weight, and in this case inches as well, is considered the comparatively easy bit – although if you have completed this 28-Day Plan you will have certainly proved to yourself that you can also be well organised and determined if you put your mind to it! However, maintaining your new figure is often much more difficult, though, as I have mentioned before, my Hip and Thigh dieters found it easy to maintain their new trim figures in the long term because they didn't feel they had really been on a 'diet' as such. While my New Inch Loss Plan has been slightly more restrictive in some respects, it has still given the slimmer considerable freedom within the realms of low-fat eating. This will stand you in good stead and it should be easy from now on to work out your own menus from the following guidelines.

You now find yourself in the delightful situation of knowing that if you want to have the occasional indulgence, such as a cream cake on someone's birthday, or an Indian meal in a restaurant, you can. An extra egg from time to time or the occasional addition of low-fat hard cheese to your menu range will give you increased flexibility when compiling your menus. In fact, you can now eat anything you like, providing it is reasonably low in fat and included as part of your meals. I think you

should still observe the rule of not eating between meals as this is the main reason for putting on weight. We can always find a little corner to fill, can't we? The discipline of eating really well, three times a day isn't too much to ask of anyone and it is much better for us.

On most diets the metabolic rate can fall because the body adjusts to a reduced calorie intake, and when people return to 'normal' eating the weight often piles back on even though they are not overeating. It all seems so unfair. The problem is less likely to occur with this New Inch Loss Plan and my other diets, because they offer so much more food than most other diets. We now know that we can still lose weight if we eat a higher proportion of carbohydrate calories compared with fat calories. This is the secret of the success of low-fat diets. Carbohydrates burn more easily, whereas fats are more easily stored. Our metabolic rate is less likely to fall, because we are not eating too little food, just far fewer fat calories. Ounce for ounce, we can eat twice as much carbohydrate food as fatty food because it contains half the number of calories!

We lose weight when we consume fewer calories than our bodies use and we make up the deficit from our stores of fat – fat that was placed there by the fat that we have eaten in the past. After reaching our desired weight, we need to

feed our bodies sufficient calories to maintain that new weight but not ruin all our good work by going back to our old high-fat eating habits, otherwise the fat will once again be deposited on our bodies! So, if we want to stay lean forever we must accept that high-fat eating is a thing of the past.

Having said that, we don't need to get paranoid about it. If in general terms you attempt to maintain a low-fat diet for life, you really should not regain your lost fat. We do need some fat in our diet to be healthy, but it should never be more than 70 grams a day on a maintenance programme.

Personally, I do not recommend that you start totting up your daily intake of grams of fat. It is a negative, time-consuming habit. Also, try to avoid the restrictive practice of calorie counting. However, calories do count, and just by not eating fat but eating lots of foods that are low in fat, you won't automatically stay slim. Don't think to yourself, 'boiled sweets don't contain fat so I can have loads of those'. If you ate them frequently on top of your normal daily intake of food, you would definitely gain weight. But if you follow the basic principles already learned on the diet, you really have nothing to fear. It is only when you start breaking the rules about forbidden foods on a regular basis that you will undo the good results that you have achieved.

The very fact that we have avoided the need to count any form of units or calories throughout the diet has weaned us away from this negative habit. It would be a shame to start now by counting fat grams. So relax and just remember what you've learned so far. Use the Fat Tables detailed on pages 194–198 as a general guide when selecting your foods.

Remember, it will be much easier to maintain your new weight if you continue to take regular exercise. Try to exercise 5 times a week for 30 minutes. You can continue to do the exercises from Week 4 of the programme 5 days a week, or you can combine the exercises with other activities that you enjoy, such as brisk walking, cycling, attending a fitness class, working out to a fitness video, and so on. Try to be as active as possible in your everyday life.

The following lists of foods and recommendations should form the pattern of foods consumed for a healthy diet. A daily diet made up of reasonable quantities from each category will ensure a balanced consumption of essential nutrients to maintain health and energy, without including unnecessary foods which add surplus calories and lead to unwanted fat. A diet which follows these recommendations will encourage a healthy digestion and increased vitality.

Protein and Minerals

A minimum of 175g (6oz) of meat, fish, eggs or cheese should be consumed daily.

450ml (¾ pint) skimmed or semi-skimmed milk should be consumed daily – maximum 600ml (1 pint) per day.

Fish	Any type	Steamed, grilled or microwaved without fat
Meat	Any type, lean cuts only	Grilled, roasted or microwaved, without fat, and with all fat trimmed off before cooking or trimmed afterwards
Poultry	Any type	Grilled, roasted or microwaved, without fat. Do not eat any skin or fat
Offal	Any type	Steamed, baked or microwaved, without fat
Eggs		Cook in any way without the use of fat. Consume no more than 4 per week
Cheese	Low-fat Cheddar	In moderation
Cheese	Cottage	Unlimited quantities may be consumed
Yogurt	Any type	Unlimited

Fruit and Vegetables

Eat 5 helpings a day.

Vegetables	Any type	Unlimited but always without butter
Fruit	Any type	Unlimited. Serve on its own, or with fromage frais or yogurt

Carbohydrates

Eat some carbohydrates at every meal.

Bread	Wholemeal or crispbreads	Unlimited if eaten without fat, otherwise limit consumption to 3 slices of bread or 8 crispbreads a day
Cereal	Breakfast	25–50g (1–2oz) per day
Rice	Brown	75g (3oz) per serving (dry weight)
Pasta	Wholemeal	Average portion 50–75g (2–3oz) dry weight
Potatoes	Boiled or baked	Unlimited if eaten without fat

Fats

Consume as little as possible.

Low-fat spread		5% low-fat spread in moderation
Cream	Single	25–50g (1–2oz) very occasionally. Use Greek yogurt instead

In addition the following foods may be eaten in moderation

Cakes made without fat

Cauliflower cheese made with low-fat cheese and skimmed milk

Horlicks, Ovaltine or Drinking Chocolate – choose low-fat brands

Ice-cream – not Cornish

Milk puddings made with skimmed milk or semi-skimmed milk

Nuts – only very few and avoid Brazils, Barcelona nuts and almonds

Pancakes made with skimmed milk

Reduced-oil salad dressing, e.g. Waistline or Weight Watchers from Heinz

Sauces, if possible made with skimmed milk, but NO butter

Yorkshire pudding made with skimmed milk in a non-stick baking tin

Sausages, if grilled well and low fat

Soups except cream soups

Soya

Trifle made with only fat-free sponge and custard made with skimmed milk – no cream

Avoid the following foods

Avocados

Biscuits, all sweet varieties

Brazil nuts, almonds, Barcelona nuts

Butter, margarine, Flora or similar products

Cakes, all except fat-free recipes

Channel Islands milk

Chapatis made with fat

Cheese, all types except Edam, cottage, low-fat Cheddar

Cheese spread

Chocolate, toffees, fudge, caramel, butterscotch

Cream, double, whipping, sterilised, tinned

Desiccated coconut

Fat from meat, streaky bacon

Fish in oil

French dressing made with oil

Fried foods, including fried bread, fried fish, fried mushrooms and fried onions etc.

Oil, lard, dripping etc.

Quiches, Scotch eggs, cheese soufflé, Welsh Rarebit etc.

Salami, pâté, pork pie, meat pies etc.

Skin from chicken, turkey, duck, goose etc.

Sprats or whitebait, fried

Marzipan

Mayonnaise

Pastries

Pork scratchings

Readers' Letters

Over the past ten years I have received thousands of letters from my readers telling me about their dieting experiences. A selection of extracts from these appears at the end of this chapter. Included in some of those letters have been a variety of questions, and in anticipation that readers of my New Inch Loss Plan may have similar ones, I am answering the most common ones here.

Questions and Answers

Q I can't eat dairy products such as milk, yogurt or cottage cheese. Does it matter if I just leave these out of the diet?

A As these foods are rich sources of calcium it would be necessary for you to take a calcium supplement if you eliminated them entirely from your diet. These foods also contain protein, but if you eat protein in other forms, e. g. fish, poultry, meat, beans etc. your diet is unlikely to be deficient. For advice about a suitable calcium supplement, consult your doctor or your local pharmacist.

Q I really hate skimmed milk but I do want to follow the diet. Are there any alternatives?

A I have to admit I don't enjoy skimmed milk either, so I use semi-skimmed milk which tastes much better.

Q I have been taking Evening Primrose Oil to help my PMT symptoms. Can I still take it while following this diet?

A If you follow the diet strictly in every other way you should still see a significant result, despite your taking EPO. However, after following the programme for 28 days, you may find that your PMT symptoms subside anyway because of the reduction in your fat intake. Many women have reported this benefit after following my diets. If this happens, you may then be able to eliminate or at least cut down your consumption of EPO.

Q I take cod liver oil capsules for my arthritis. Will the diet still work for me?

A The answer to this question is similar to the last one. The diet will still work despite the high fat content of the capsules, because you will be reducing your overall intake of fats dramatically. Benefits in inch and weight loss should still be apparent. The other good news is that many who have followed my low-fat diets have also enjoyed significant improvements in their arthritic condition. Their level of pain reduced, and their mobility increased, so you too may find in time that the cod liver oil can be cut down.

Q I can't eat breakfast. Is it all right if I skip just this meal because I really can't face anything first thing in the morning?

A Breakfast is important on this diet because it helps to cure evening bingeing. We often binge late in the day because psychologically we know that we are not going to eat until midday tomorrow, and our bodies start saying, 'so let's stock up now'. If eating early in the morning is inconvenient or unappetising, pack something to take with you to work, but try to eat it before 10am. If you can't bear anything major, just have a couple of pieces of fruit or a couple of diet yogurts.

Q I already go to a slimming club and I wonder if I should stop while I am on your diet?

A No. The group therapy will help you to stick with the diet and I would hope that the class leader would have no objection to you following this plan. After all, they are there to help you get slimmer. Also, if you already attend an exercise class, there is no reason for you to stop that either. In fact, there is no need to change any of the activities you do if you enjoy them. Do the New Inch Loss exercise plan as well as your class if you can.

Q I am not overweight – in fact, some would say I am underweight. From the waist upwards I suppose I am really too slim. However, I do have fat on my thighs and bottom and would dearly love to lose inches from that area without actually losing any more weight. Is there anything I can do to solve the problem?

A If you just follow the Maintenance Diet and do the exercises, you will lose inches without losing weight. This is because you will be consuming significantly less fat than before and this, in turn, will cause the fat stores that are already deposited on your body to reduce. As low-fat eating leads only to the reduction of fat, weight will not go from lean areas.

Q I am a shift worker. How can I work the diet into my abnormal daily pattern?

A If we assume you work on a weekly shift, the easiest solution is to decide on a week's menu in advance. Write it down, and from midnight prior to the first day to midnight of the 7th day, you can have 21 meals including 7 breakfasts, 7 lunches and 7 dinners, but don't feel restricted as to when you eat them. Just cross them off as you consume them. Ideally, it is better if you have your main meal before going to work, then eat your snack (lunch) meal at work and have your 'breakfast' when you return. This way you won't be going to bed on a very full stomach but should be able to sleep having had something to eat. Trial and error is the only answer, so play around with different formulas until you find one to suit you.

Q I've stuck rigidly to the diet and I've lost loads of inches, but I haven't lost much weight. I'm not complaining, but I just wondered why?

A No two people respond the same way to any diet programme and some people definitely seem to lose more weight than others. Part of the reason is that fat doesn't weigh very much – it is much lighter than muscle. However, the most important result is the loss of inches, because that's when our clothes fit more comfortably and we actually look slimmer. Recently one lady telephoned me. She had been on my low-fat diet and had been advised by a friend not to weigh herself but just to record her progress with a tape measure. In 8 weeks she had lost a total of 27in (68.5cm)! She was positively thrilled. 'So who needs scales anyway?' she said.

Q I have a problem with my back. Should I try these exercises?

A Because spinal problems can be so varied and complex it is always advisable to show the exercises in this book to your physiotherapist/chiropractor, or whoever looks after your back, before you try them. They will advise you according to your individual capabilities.

Q I've heard that muscle weighs more than fat. Is this true?

A Yes. You only need to take a piece of fat from the butcher's and compare it with a similar-sized piece of lean meat, which is almost pure muscle. The fat is much lighter in weight. This is why the reduction of fat (and therefore inches) on your body as a result of following this diet will be more significant than the actual weight you lose. The good thing is that you will only lose the very parts of you that you wish to lose – that is the fatty parts. Your muscle tissue (including your heart) should not be depleted, which is another reason why this diet is so healthy.

Q But won't the exercises build muscles and therefore cause me to gain weight?

A No. The exercises will tone your muscles but not cause them to become very large. Weightlifters build muscles by lifting very heavy weights, many, many times. Their muscles are built up to cope with this load and then put under a greater load so that they grow even more. We are not doing that in this programme, so don't worry!

Q My husband needs to lose weight? Could he do this programme?

A Yes. Men, generally speaking, tend to retain their excess fat around their abdomens. Many men have been on my low-fat diets with tremendous success. They lose their 'tums' but retain their manly figures! They should increase the quantities of food allowed by 25 per cent.

Q I like this way of eating. I feel so much better now and have much more energy. In fact, I feel I never want to return to my old high-fat eating habits. Can I stay on this low-fat diet for ever?

A Most certainly. Medical experts now unanimously agree that we should all eat less fat in our daily diet and do more exercise. Providing you have a varied, nutritious diet, it can only do you good.

Q There are certain items on the diet I like a lot – for instance, I have porridge every morning for my breakfast and salad sandwiches with wholemeal bread for my lunch. Is it OK to keep repeating the same menus?

A Providing you eat a good helping of protein for dinner (around 115–175g/4–6oz) with lots of vegetables and have a fruit dessert, it is fine. Vary your evening meal so that you get a good selection of nutrients. If you find a certain menu really suits you, by all means stick to it. Perhaps take a multivitamin and mineral tablet to make doubly sure you get all the essential vitamins and minerals on a daily basis.

Readers' Comments

Mr T. S. Roberts from Leicestershire:

Over the last few weeks, I feel I have achieved a way of eating that will remain forever. I look and feel healthier, fitter and possibly younger. Clothes, particularly trousers, are more comfortable to wear and I can now do up the top buttons on shirts. My golf is improving with 'less padding' to swing around. Also, my wife says my snoring has reduced!

After 19 weeks on the diet Mr Roberts lost 2st (12.7kg).

Mrs Jane Clements from South Africa:

I feel great and so very excited at my weight and inch loss. I bought a new skirt – not a 14, as I've been for years, but a 12. I wanted to tell the world! I'm enthusiastic, too, that it is a sensible pattern of eating for the future. Thank you.

Miss Wendy Whitehead from the West Midlands:

I have been on the diet for 11 weeks and I would like to say that this is one of the best things that has ever happened to me. I am so pleased with the results. I am 5ft 1in (1.55m) tall and was 9st 1lb (57.6kg) when I started. My measurements were: bust 38in (97cm), waist 32in (81cm), hips 37½in (95cm). They are now: bust 36in (91cm), waist 27in (69cm), hips 35in (89cm). I have also lost 2in (5cm) from the tops of my arms. I think this is wonderful. I would not have believed that I could eat so much and still lose so many inches. I feel so proud of myself. This diet is fantastic, it's true you really do feel well and healthy and I am sure you have made a lot of people very happy.

Mrs J. Kendall from Lincolnshire:

I have been on numerous diets and got fed up after 2 or 3 weeks because of lack of variety of food. Also, I did not seem to be getting any thinner. So as you can imagine I was a little pessimistic about yours. I even made a note in my diary saying the diet would have to be pretty wonderful to do anything for my hips and thighs! But it is wonderful. I have lost 1st (6.4kg), 3in (8cm) from my hips and 3in (8cm) from my widest part. I get so many compliments, it is fantastic. I did not think I could have eaten so much – it is what I call educated eating.

Mrs L. Smith from Leeds:

When I started the diet I was 10st 6 lb (66.2 kg). I am 5ft 3in (1.6m) tall. People used to say I had 'child-bearing' hips. After 5 weeks on the diet and 4 weeks maintenance, I am now 8st 8lb (54.4 kg) – a total loss of 1st 12lb (11.7kg). I lost

2in (5cm) from my waist, 4in (10cm) from my hips, 5in (12cm) from my widest part and 3in (8cm) from each leg. I cannot believe the transformation – now the lower part of my body is in proportion with the top. I have a lot more confidence and feel like going out more. When I started, I hoped for the kind of results that I read about in your book. I found I reached them within 3 weeks and this gave me the incentive to carry on.

Mrs V. Hamilton from Warwickshire:

I started your diet in March, weighing 10st (63.5 kg) and by July got down to 8st 2lb (51.7kg). On holiday in Minorca I can't tell you how pleased I was to go on the beach in a bikini with no overhanging flab on my hips and thighs. It has now become a way of life for me and I find it so easy to do. There are plenty of foods to eat, and I rarely feel hungry. I am now a size 10, which I haven't been since I was 20 years old. This diet has made me like myself a lot more. Thank you for giving me a new lease of life.

Mrs J. Garner from Grantham:

In 9 weeks I have lost 12lb (5.4 kg), 4in (10cm) from my waist and 5in (12.7cm) from my hips. In addition, I used to suffer a good deal of digestive discomfort and that is now a thing of the past. As well as feeling much fitter and more active, life is generally much more pleasant. That haggard, ill appearance so often connected with weight loss has been noticeably absent. The final bonus is that my friends say that I look radiantly fit and trim – as I am 67 this is a great compliment.

Miss N. Williams from London:

I started your diet 9 months ago; my weight was 12st 4lb (78kg). I found it so simple, easy and good sense to follow, it was like an inspiration to me. My previous dieting attempts had produced weight loss but from all the wrong places! I am now 9st 4lb (59kg), 3st (19kg) lighter, hips were 45in (114cm) now 38in (97cm), bust was 36in (91cm) now 34 (86cm), waist was 29½in (75cm) now 26in (66cm) and my biggest claim to fame is that I now wear size 10 jeans! I cannot thank you enough for completely re-educating my attitude towards food. People keep commenting on how well I look. I feel proud of myself again.

Mrs J. W. from Nottingham:

After losing 23lb (10.4kg), 4in (10cm) off waist, 4in (10cm) off left thigh, 3in (8cm) off right thigh, Mrs J. W. wrote:

It's been great to chew foods! Sachets are boring. It's not really a diet but a new healthy and great way of eating – and for life, not just a few weeks of the year.

Mrs J. Warner from West Yorkshire:

All my life I have tried various ways and diets to lose weight, but to no avail. My legs from my hips down were like tree trunks. I got a terrible nickname, when young, very embarrassing and undermining. I just felt I wasn't wanted with the rest of the girls, treated like someone who had the plague. Having read your book, I thought: now I'm going to get somewhere. I have gone from 11st 4lb (71.6kg) to 9st 8lb (60.7kg) at almost 63 years of age! I think it's incredible, I'm so thrilled I just can't believe it. My figure is better now than it has ever been. You have done me a power of good in more ways than one and boosted my morale tremendously. A slim person always looks lovely and has the very best advantages in life. They feel more confident and relaxed.

Mr N. Vernon from Cheshire:

I am indebted to you for the diet and resultant success in my case. I am 49, and for as long as I can remember I have been overweight at between 13½–14st (82.5–92kg), the most I have ever lost on a diet being 7lb–1st (3.1–6.3kg) and that was with great difficulty. I started your diet in January when I was 14st 5lb (91kg) with a 44in (112cm) waist. Today (June) I am now 11st (70kg) exactly, with a waist of 36in (91cm). I am now wearing clothes that I have had for donkey's years but could not get into. What I love about your diet is that the motivation to continue is automatic and enjoyable.

Mrs D. Langley from York:

After following your diet, I'm delighted my weight has remained stable. I can honestly say I am still enjoying sticking to the diet, for it is so easy and very rewarding. You can use any of my quotes if it will help others to gain as much happiness and confidence as I myself have done.

Mrs F. Kirkman from Leicestershire:

I'm amazed with the diet and myself! My weight was 10st 2lb (64.4kg) and is now 9st 4lb (59kg). My left thigh was 23in (58cm) and is now 21in (53cm) and my right thigh was 22in (56cm) and is now 20in (50cm). It doesn't sound much on paper but it really is fantastic. I have lost over 4in (10cm) off my hips! My husband has been very supportive, I have had lots of lovely remarks and have treated myself to a shaped skirt which, previously, I wouldn't have bought. I don't really feel as though I have been on a diet as such but a re-educated course in healthy eating. I can see the massive improvements this diet has made to how I look and feel.

Mrs S. Beers from Nottinghamshire:

My husband encouraged me to buy your diet book, but frankly I was so sceptical. I could not believe I could lose the fat. All my fat seemed to have accumulated around my waist. Tight clothes made me look 3 months pregnant. I've lost 14lb (6.3kg) and 4in (10cm) off my waist! I can now wear straight skirts with confidence. Previous diets have left me scraggy and flat-chested. I have always been very active and had plenty of energy, but it is a lot easier when you are lighter – you also look better and I feel so much more confident now.

Mrs D. B. from Newport:

I was fed up with people saying, 'you're not fat, why do you want to diet?' But the fact is I was flabby and felt fat, especially around the hips and thighs. After a week on the diet and losing 5lb (2.2kg) and 1½in (4cm) off my hips I can feel and see a difference.

Mrs A. Jones from Leicester:

A very big thank you for letting me into the secret of losing inches and weight without starving. I have been on the diet for 10 weeks and have lost 25lb (11.3kg), 5in (12.7cm) from my hips and 4in (10cm) from my widest part, plus 2in (5cm) off each leg. I intend to carry on to see if I can get into size 12 clothes, already having achieved size 14 trousers, which hasn't happened for at least 15 years. Also, since I've been on the diet my indigestion has gone which is another big advantage.

Mrs S. F. from Warwick:

I have lost 14lb (6.3kg), including 5in (12.7cm) off the top of my legs. I feel absolutely marvellous, and everyone compliments me on my new image. I even purchased my very first straight skirt last week and it is a size 10. I am so pleased and grateful and cannot thank you enough for what you have done for me.

A chartered surveyor who wishes to remain anonymous wrote:

I feel I must drop you a line to proclaim yet another benefit, or side-effect of your diet. Some 8 weeks ago, a sceptical, overweight, middle-aged male joined his wife on the diet and at the same time stopped excessive alcohol consumption. A weight loss in the first week of some 5lb (2.2kg) followed by 3lb (1.4kg) and since then an average 2lb (0.9kg) per week has turned the sceptic into a believer who now feels very much fitter and whose eyesight has improved enormously. I regularly have to measure floor-to-ceiling heights and at one time could no longer read my tape at anything over 8ft (2.5m). Now it is relatively easy to read at 10ft (3m).

Mrs J. T. from Essex:

After reading some of the success stories, I found myself close to tears, as I know what the success must mean to the people who have written about them. I am 26 and all my adult life – and probably most of my childhood too – I have been overweight, until now. I began by planning a fortnight's menu, and haven't looked back. To date I have lost 2st 10lb (17.2kg). I've lost over 7in (18cm) off the top of my legs. Everyone has commented on the dramatic change and I'm becoming more confident day by day. How can anyone describe the relief of being a reasonable size and of no longer being fat? Every part of me is smaller, I've got cheekbones! and part of my relief in losing so much weight is that it means I'm now treating the body God put me in with much more respect.

Jacqueline Storey from North Yorkshire:

I was a very unhappy person. I didn't like to go out with my fiancé, and over Christmas when we went to visit my parents I refused to go out with them. I felt self-conscious. I wasn't outrageously huge, I was fat. I weighed 13st 8lb (86.1kg). My measurements were 40in (102cm), 32in (81cm), 46in (117cm). In January I decided I was going to slim down to 10st (63.5kg). In May I reached my target but will continue with the diet or 'changed eating habits' as I like to call it. The results are absolutely stunning. I feel so much better, not just physically but emotionally too. I feel so much more confident and now enjoy going out at weekends with my fiancé. I am wearing skirts and trousers that have been redundant in my wardrobe since before I met my fiancé. My new measurements are 35in (89cm), 26in (66cm), 39in (99cm). Total weight loss 3st (19kg). Never again will I go back to old, unhealthy and gluttonous eating habits.

Mrs W. P. from Buckinghamshire:

My husband went to the Falklands in the last week of January, so I decided that during his 4-month tour away I would shed my excess pounds. On 30 January my measurements were 35in (89cm), 29in (74cm) 40in (102cm) and I weighed 11st 4 lb (71.6kg). The night before my husband was due back I measured 34in (86cm), 25in (64cm) 34½in (88cm) and weighed 9st 8lb (60.9kg)! When I met him at the airport, he didn't recognise me for a while, then was totally amazed I'd lost weight from where it mattered most on me – my hips and thighs. Now I feel so much healthier and fitter.

Mrs M. S. Robson from Birmingham:

After losing my husband 3 years ago and last year losing my lovely mum, I turned to eating for comfort almost non-stop. I went from 7st 7lb (47.6kg) to 8st 12lb (56.2kg) and being so small (5ft 1in) I felt like a fat pig. After 3 weeks on the diet I have already lost 6lb (2.7kg). Diets have always made me look haggard before, but not this one. I feel fit and healthy. Also, as I have a spastic colon, I have found the high fibre a great help and all my pain has now gone.

Grams per 25g/1oz (approx.)

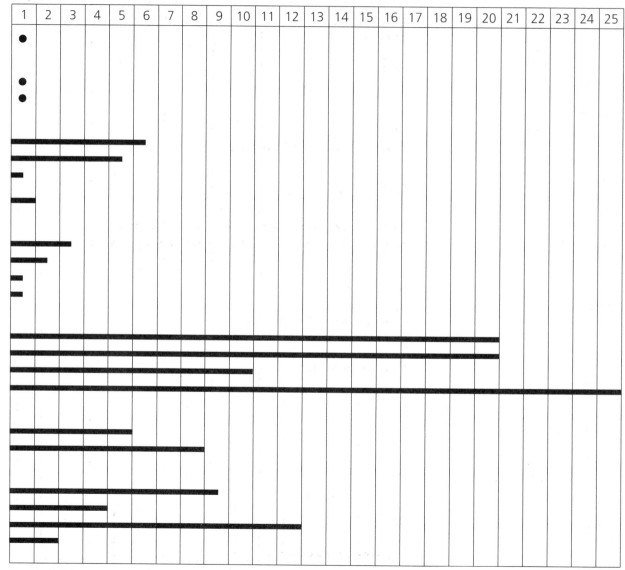

	1	2	3	4	5	6	7	8	9	10	11	12	13	14	15	16	17	18	19	20	21	22	23	24	25

Alcohol

Beans
Baked
Kidney

Biscuits
Sweet
Savoury
Rye

Bread

Breakfast cereal
Muesli type
Porridge (dry)
Flakes – corn or bran
Weetabix

Fats and oils
Butter and margarine
Flora
Low-fat spread
Oil – all types

Cakes
Cakes – average
Pastry – average

Cheese
Ordinary Cheddar
Low-fat brands
Cream cheese
Low-fat soft cheese

● = negligible

Grams per 25g/1oz (approx.)

Food	Fat (grams per 25g/1oz approx.)
Fromage frais	2
Low-fat fromage frais	negligible
Cottage cheese	negligible
Quark – low fat	negligible
Confectionery	
Sweets – boiled/mint	negligible
Chocolate	8
Cream	
Single	5
Whipping	9
Double	12
Cornish clotted	15
Eggs	
Whole	3
White only	negligible
Yolk only	8
Fish	
Oily fish*	5
White fish	1
Flour	
All types – average	1
Grains	
All types – average	1
Fruit	
Most types	negligible
Exceptions:	
Avocado	7

● = negligible   *Although oily fish is relatively high in fat, it contains valuable nutrients which should be included in a low-fat diet.

Grams per 25g/1oz (approx.)

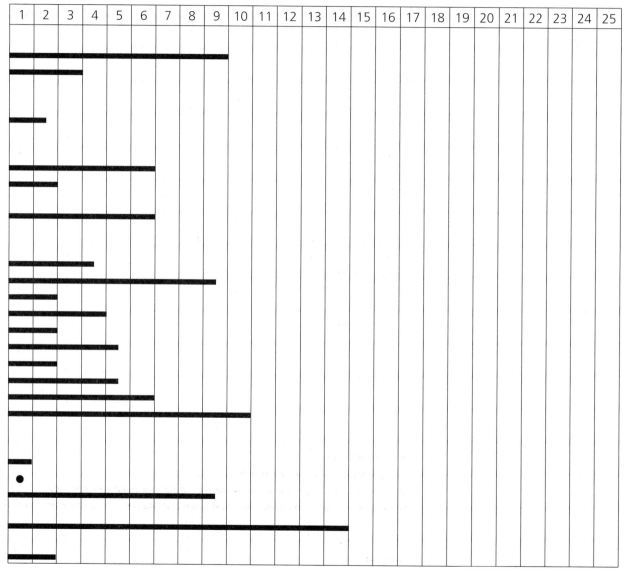

| | 1 | 2 | 3 | 4 | 5 | 6 | 7 | 8 | 9 | 10 | 11 | 12 | 13 | 14 | 15 | 16 | 17 | 18 | 19 | 20 | 21 | 22 | 23 | 24 | 25 |

Fruit continued
Coconut flesh
Olives

Game
Roast – without skin

Ice cream
Choc ice
Plain

Marzipan

Meat
Bacon – lean only
Bacon – lean & fat
Beef – lean only
Beef – lean & fat
Lamb – lean only
Lamb – lean & fat
Pork – lean only
Pork – lean & fat
Sausages – average
Salami

Milk
Fresh
Skimmed
Coffee whitener

Nuts – average

Offal – average

● = negligible

Grams per 25g/1oz (approx.)

Food	Fat (grams per 25g/1oz)
Pasta – average	negligible
Pickles	negligible
Poultry	
Chicken – light meat – no skin	1
Chicken – dark meat – no skin	2
Duck – meat only – no skin	3
Turkey – light meat	negligible
Turkey – dark meat	1
Puddings	
Cheesecake	9
Christmas pudding	4
Fruit pie	5
Jelly	negligible
Meringues	negligible
Pancakes	5
Trifle	2
Pulses & lentils	negligible
Rice	negligible
Sauces	
Reduced-oil dressing	4
Salad cream	8
Mayonnaise	16
French dressing	20
Tomato ketchup	negligible
Soups – average	2

● = negligible

Grams per 25g/1oz (approx.)

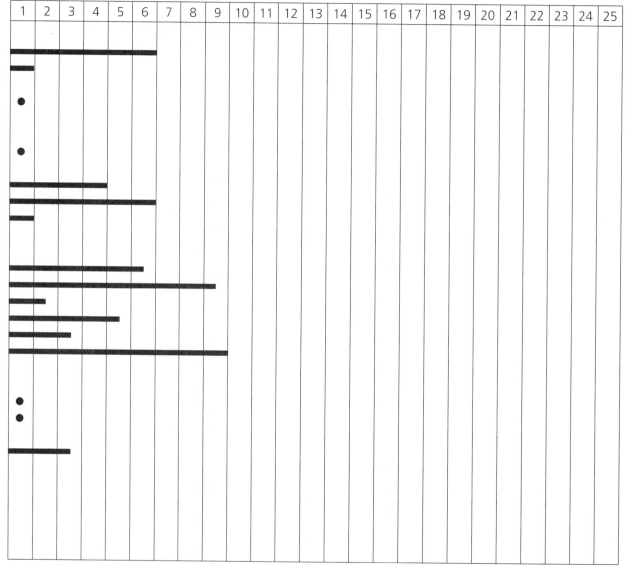

	1	2	3	4	5	6	7	8	9	10	11	12	13	14	15	16	17	18	19	20	21	22	23	24	25

Soya
Full fat
Low fat

Sugar

Vegetables
Most (including potatoes)
Exceptions:
   Ackee
   Avocado
   Green mung beans

Vegetables – cooked with fat
Fried mushrooms
Fried onions
Potatoes – roast with fat
Potatoes – chips (frozen & fried)
Oven chips – frozen
Crisps

Yogurt
Most low-fat brands
French style set yogurt

Yorkshire pudding

● = negligible

Tangible Goals

	Target Date	Date Achieved
Short Term		
Long Term		
Ultimate Goal		

Intangible Goals

	Target Date	Date Achieved
Short Term		
Long Term		
Ultimate Goal		

WEIGHT AND INCH LOSS RECORD CHART

DATE:														**Total loss**
Weight														
Total weight lost to date														
Bust	39													
Waist	35													
Widest part	35/39													
Hips	43													
L. Thigh	26													
R. Thigh	26													
L. Knee	16													
R. Knee	17													
L. Arm	14													
R. Arm	14													
Total inches lost this week														
Total to date														